MY BEEF WITH MEAT

The Healthiest Argument for Eating a Plant-Strong Diet— Plus 140 New Engine 2 Recipes

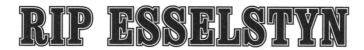

RIP ESSELSTYN

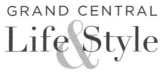

GRAND CENTRAL
Life & Style

NEW YORK · BOSTON

Engine 2 and Plant-Strong are registered trademarks of Engine 2 For Life, LLC

Copyright © 2013 by Rip Esselstyn

Grand Central Life & Style
Hachette Book Group
237 Park Avenue
New York, NY 10017

www.GrandCentralLifeandStyle.com

Printed in the United States of America

RRD-C

First Edition: May 2013
10 9 8 7 6 5 4 3 2 1

Grand Central Life & Style is an imprint of Grand Central Publishing. The Grand Central Life & Style name and logo are trademarks of Hachette Book Group, Inc.

The Hachette Speakers Bureau provides a wide range of authors for speaking events. To find out more, go to www.HachetteSpeakersBureau.com or call (866) 376-6591.

Library of Congress Cataloging-in-Publication Data has been applied for.

To my parents, Ann and Essy.
You made this possible. I love you.

Contents

PART II
THE RECIPES

Introduction

Forty-two-year-old Nick Gravina was one of the fittest firefighters in the South Metro, Colorado, fire department. He was also a total beast at the Firefighter Combat Challenge, a timed competition that involves climbing a 50-foot tower with five flights of stairs carrying a 42-pound roll of fire hose, descending and slamming a sledgehammer into a 160-pound metal beam until it moves 5 feet, pulling a charged hose line 75 feet, opening the nozzle and flowing water and hitting a target, and dragging a 175-pound dummy 106 feet to the finish line. Nick was able to do all this in less than 1 minute and 35 seconds, all the while wearing full gear and breathing air from a 30-pound Air-Pak on his back!

But I didn't meet Nick in an athletic contest. We met because Nick's mother sent me an e-mail asking for help.

Although Nick's athletic abilities were amazing, his health wasn't. One day in March 2012, Nick, who is married and has two young kids, started to feel some chest pain that he thought was just a bad case of indigestion, but it was painful enough that he alerted his crew, who immediately hooked him up to the heart monitor to get a look at his heart. The paramedic saw an abnormal rhythm and called an ambulance just as Nick's heart stopped beating and he stopped breathing—he was, basically, dead. The firefighters immediately gave Nick two defibrillation shocks but they didn't work. So the crew started CPR, and Nick's heart barely began to beat on its own again. The ambulance then rushed him to the hospital, where for the next hour Nick went in and out of cardiac arrest while his crew and doctors tried desperately to save his life. After one hour of CPR and eighteen shocks to his heart, Nick's doctors finally were able to remove a blood clot from his heart, saving his life.

When Nick recovered, he was determined to do everything in his power to make sure this attack was a onetime event. He was a great athlete, but he'd always eaten whatever he wanted, thinking he could burn everything off since he was so fit. Then his mother sent him a copy of my book, *The Engine 2 Diet*, which lured him into the plant-strong life.

Since going on the E2 diet, Nick's total cholesterol has come down to 83 mg/dl, his LDL is 35 mg/dl, he's leaner than he's ever been, and he feels empowered with the knowledge that he and his food choices now control his health destiny. He is now a dedicated E2er. Way to go, Nick!

Nick isn't alone. All over the country people are learning about healthy plant-based diets. In fact, things have changed dramatically since my first book, *The Engine 2 Diet*, was published in February of 2009. People are waking up to the fact that the current paradigm is broken. The answer is not another pill, procedure, or doctor, or more legislation. Unbelievably, the answer is right in front of our faces. But we've been blind because we had no idea the answer could be so simple. It's like Glinda, the good witch of the North, telling Dorothy she's always had the power to leave Oz and go home—all she ever had to do was click her heels together three times and say, "There's no place like home."

It's the same with eating a plant-strong diet and the wonders it can do to prevent and reverse disease. Say it three times (and click your heels if you'd like): "There's no diet like a plant-based diet."

Over the last decade more and more people are figuring this out. The plant-strong boom is on! High-profile celebrities from television hosts Ellen DeGeneres and Rosie O'Donnell to NFL star running back Arian Foster, from actress Michelle Pfeiffer to President Bill Clinton have joined the plant-based team. Books and documentaries on the subject are selling like plant-based hotcakes—especially the documentary *Forks Over Knives* (starring T. Colin Campbell, Ph.D., author of *The China Study*, and my father, Caldwell B. Esselstyn Jr., M.D., author of *Prevent and Reverse Heart Disease*), which has become one of the top-selling and most viewed documentaries in America for the last two years.

Other parts of America are noticing too, from nutritionists to doctors, from restaurants to stores. In 2010, the natural food supermarket chain Whole Foods Market launched its healthy eating initiative to educate the company's thousands of employees and millions of customers about the benefits of eating a whole-food, plant-strong, nutrient-dense, healthy-fat diet. CEO John Mackey invited me to help the company do this, and so after twelve years at the Austin Fire Department, I jumped off the fire engine and stepped out of my bunker gear to rescue people from food instead of fires.

And yet, despite this terrific momentum, too many people are still eating terribly, and too many people are ill-informed about food. In fact, even after Nick's heart attack and brush with death, his fellow firefighters still can't understand why he doesn't eat meat or drink milk.

That's why Nick's mother called me—to ask me to support his new, lifesaving diet, but also to give him the information he needs to win over his firefighting friends. We talked for more than an hour, and I gave him all the ammunition he needed to win every argument his fellow firefighters might throw at him.

That's exactly what this book does as well. Inside are all the facts you'll need to combat the silly claims and misguided myths you'll hear from naysayers who throw out statements like "You can't get enough protein eating plants," or "You can't get enough vitamins," and so on. You'll learn the truth about protein, the facts about vitamins, and the myths about meat. In fact, by the time you've finished this book, you'll be an expert on everything you need to know to win any argument with a meat eater. And you'll be more convinced than ever that your plant-based diet rules!

Of course, once you've won the argument with your words, you'll want to win it with your cooking as well. To that end, I'm offering you 140 mouthwatering Engine 2 recipes to serve to your no-longer-doubtful friends. These recipes will put a smile on your decreasing belly and you'll be able to wow your friends at breakfast with Savory Shiitake and Cheesy Oats (p. 139), Zeb's Waffles (p. 144), and Cranberry-Polenta French Toast (p. 147); at lunch with Asparagus and Cream of Cashew Collard Wraps (p. 151), Armadillo Sweet Potatoes (p. 156), and Rockin' Reuben on Rye (p. 168); at dinner with BBQ LOL (Lentil Oat Loaf) (p. 176), Summer Soba (p. 196), and Raise-the-Barn Butternut Squash–Vegetable Lasagna (p. 199); and for dessert with Bittersweet Chocolate Truffles (p. 264), Banana-Oatmeal Peanut Butter Cookies (p. 259), and Mango-Cherry "Ice Cream" (p. 256). You'll find recipes for the soup lovers in your circle, as well as the burger and fries fans. You'll even find sauces, dips, salads, and salsas.

To source these recipes, I talked not only to my family, where everyone has been collecting plant-strong recipes for years, but to Engine 2 fans all over the country. Some of these people are professional chefs such as John Mercer, Fran Costigan, and Lindsay Nixon; some are parents such as Maria Steiner and Renee Van de Motter; some are working professionals such as Polly LaBarre, Wendy Solganik, and Dick

DuBois. What they all have in common is they're all eating plant-strong and creating a new arsenal of amazing recipes that are plant based, filled with whole foods, and always delicious.

Armed with these facts and recipes, you, like Nick and millions of others, will be on your way to revolutionizing the way you eat and the way you live. An E2 plant-strong diet can rescue your health and save your life. There's no argument there!

Stay Connected with Engine 2!

For more information about *My Beef with Meat*, please go to mybeefwithmeat.com—and if you have any questions about science, the recipes, or anything else, let me know! Also, check out our Engine 2 site, engine2.com, for tons of resources, recipes, videos, and everything else to get you started with your plant-strong life! Look at Engine 2 Extra as well—here we have a wonderful support network available with coaching and information on our daily 28-day challenges (engine2extra.com).

Like us on Facebook! We have a great community with loads of plant-strong tips (www.facebook.com/Engine2Diet). Find us on Pinterest, where there are hundreds of recipes, articles, and plant-strong finds pinned on pinterest boards (pinterest.com/engine2diet). Don't forget to follow us on Twitter too (@engine2diet)! Ask questions, post photos, and tag us! Join up for occasional Twitter chats as well! And check us out on Instagram: tag us and show us your plant-strong meals, places where you find E2 products, etc. (instagram.com/engine2diet).

Don't forget to come to an event! Join us for our Farms 2 Forks events held across the country (www.farms2forks.com). And finally, check out our new food line with lots of delicious and easy-to-prepare plant-strong meals: www.wholefoodsmarket.com/engine2.

PART I

THE FACTS

Let's begin with The Facts—thirty-six of them! If you've been following the Engine 2 diet, or you've just been adding a lot of fruits and vegetables to your diet, you probably can't count how many times you've heard naysayers proclaim, "Meat, it's what's for dinner" or, "Milk—it does a body good." And how many times have you heard people make fun of your plant-based diet and spout their so-called facts about why you need to eat red meat, chicken, fish, and dairy. The real fact is: Their facts *aren't* facts! They're myths!

The unfortunate reality is that the powerful meat and dairy lobbies have been successfully spreading their propaganda for many decades. The fortunate reality is that we are now in the midst of the greatest information era in the history of mankind and the truth about food and nutrition and good health is rising up and resonating with people around the world. Why? Because the answer is so simple: Plants can heal. Plants can nourish. Plants can nurture. Plants can give you everything you need to be the healthiest person you can be and live the life you deserve to live.

So it's time to learn the real truth. Not only that, when you're done with these chapters, you'll be fully equipped to outwit, outsmart, and outmaneuver all those meat-loving and plant-fearing souls you come across day after day.

Join me in a plant-strong healthy eating revolution. Let's become a nation of responsible eaters. Let's learn the truth about nutrition! Bring on the facts! Go plant-strong!

1

Animal Protein Is Dead Wrong

The classic fallback argument of meat eaters and milk-mustache devotees is that a plant-based diet will make you chronically sick—and sickly looking as well. They also insist that eating all that animal protein helps them ward off the flu and protects against heart attack, stroke, and cancer, right?

Well, these people couldn't be more wrong. It's not the plant-based foods that will make you ill, it's the meat and the liquid meat (i.e.: dairy) that can lead to sickness and death. Consider this: If your food had a face or a mother (or comes from something that did), then it also has varying amounts of artery-clogging, plaque-plugging, and cholesterol-hiking animal protein, animal cholesterol, and animal fat. These substances are the building blocks of the chronic diseases that plague Western society.

Surprised? Americans have become so accustomed to chronic illness that we simply assume that conditions such as heart disease or stroke are like wrinkles—bound to happen eventually and a natural part of the aging process. They are certainly common. Just look at the explosion of new blood pressure and cholesterol drugs in recent years; doctors and pharmacies seem to be giving them out like candy.

According to the *Harvard Health Letter*, in 2011 more than 32 million Americans were taking statins for high cholesterol. And a 2010 report by the Centers for Disease Control (CDC) found that nearly *half* of all Americans use some kind of prescription drugs on a regular basis.

Yet despite our attempts to medicate away our misery, Americans are sicker than ever. According to the CDC, in 2005 133 million Americans—nearly one out of every two adults—had at least one chronic illness.

And the percentage of middle-aged Americans suffering from three or more ailments has almost doubled in the last fifteen years.

It doesn't really look like all those medications are doing a good job. And it's no surprise. All of these drugs—whether it's statins for high cholesterol, beta blockers for high blood pressure, glucophage for high blood sugar, or acetaminophen for inflammation—are doing nothing at all to address the root cause of the problems they're supposed to treat.

Doctors who prescribe such medications are myopically addressing only the symptoms of disease, making our numbers look good and giving people a false sense of security. The truth is, all of these ailments can result from lifestyle choices about food. Period. So tell these meat eaters to stop thinking they are an exception to this rule!

Here's where some people step in and say: "But chronic ailments like heart disease, stroke, and diabetes are mostly hereditary! If both your grandfathers had heart problems, you probably will too, right?"

Not necessarily. One such person was Mickey Mantle. Arguably the best pure hitter in the history of baseball, the Mick swore he wouldn't live past the age of fifty because most of the men in his family had died from Hodgkin's disease (a cancer of the lymph tissue). So he lived hard, drank heavily, ate poorly, and ended up dying at the age of 63—not from cancer but alcohol-induced cirrhosis of the liver. (He never did come down with Hodgkin's.) Nearing his final days, he said: "If I'd known I was gonna live this long, I'd have taken a lot better care of myself."

Many of the ailments that slow us down, weaken our bones, or strangle our heart are completely avoidable, whether or not your ancestors had them—and not by taking drugs. Your blood pressure doesn't have to be high, your bones don't have to crumble, and your arteries don't have to clog! Most chronic diseases, no matter how many undesirable chromosome mutations we may have, can be avoided by controlling what goes into our body.

Consider that the National Heart, Lung, and Blood Institute recently completed a ten-year study, concluding that nearly all males over age 60 and all females over age 70 reared on a typical Western, animal-based diet are already suffering from heart disease and should be treated as such. Even more frightening: In almost 50 percent of heart attacks, the first symptom is instant death.

What is at the core of this terrible disease? Plaque. Plaque is a waxy, fatty deposit that can build up in various places in the body, including the inside of the arteries, the blood vessels that carry blood away from the heart. Over time, plaque grows even greasier, more fatty, and nastier, and can become so thick that it severely constricts the flow of blood. If left untreated—or worse, if the unhealthy diet that promoted plaque in the first place persists—the arteries may become completely closed off, triggering a heart attack.

While blood thinners can increase the flow of blood, and medications like nitroglycerin can even temporarily dilate the arteries to prevent death, your fork is the only tool that can actually help *reverse* the buildup of plaque in your system.

Surprisingly, artery blockage causes less than 10 percent of heart attacks. The cause of nearly 90 percent of them is gel plaques, similar to small pimples that line the arterial wall. When one decides to pop, your body forms a blood clot. The result, more often than not, is no blood flow downstream to the heart. Ouch!

This is how newscaster Tim Russert died. He had perfect blood pressure and cholesterol numbers (thanks in part to the titanic amount of medication he was taking on a daily basis). In addition, his doctors had recently given him a clean bill of health. Yet two weeks later, a gel plaque burst in his body.

Sadly, he is not the exception to the rule. This is happening all over America every single day. And here is the crazy, crazy, crazy thing: All of the statin drugs that almost 32 million Americans take daily do almost zilch, zero, nada, to prevent gel plaques from rupturing.

If you take a close look at the NNT, or numbers needed to treat, for people taking a given medication to get a positive result, you'll find that 100 people need to be taking a statin drug for 1 person to be helped. 100 to 1! That is an egregiously poor track record. The only subgroup of people who modestly benefit from taking a statin drug are those who have had a prior cardiovascular event.

So if your doctor is worth his or her salt, he or she should tell you these statistics before placing you on a statin drug. The doctor should also inform you of the laundry list of known side effects from statins, including fatigue, muscle aches, depression, headaches, difficulty sleeping, flushing, drowsiness, dizziness, nausea and/or vomiting, abdominal cramping and/or pain, bloating and/or gas, diarrhea, constipation, rashes, impotence, diabetes, and cognitive issues such as forgetfulness and confusion—to name a few.

Lifelong cigarette smokers don't get their wind back by switching to cigars; for their lungs to regenerate, they have to quit altogether. The same goes for your arteries. Taking a pill then continuing to eat meat won't help you.

In fact, my father (a surgeon and an expert on cardiac disease) is convinced that people have the profound ability to destroy these Darth Vader death-star gel plaques using only their forks—by eating whole, plant-healing foods—in as little as three weeks! Try that one on for size: Three weeks to make yourself heart attack proof!

So if you want to glow with health, then ditch the animals and bring on the plants. After all, the largest organization of food and nutrition professionals in the United States, the Academy of Nutrition and Dietetics (AND), says that "appropriately planned vegetarian diets, including total vegetarian or vegan diets, are healthful, nutritionally adequate and may provide health benefits in the prevention and treatment of certain diseases." Also, a 2009 report by the AND noted that eaters of plant-based diets low in saturated fat and cholesterol "tend to have a lower body mass index and lower overall cancer rates."

Translation: Plants are the bomb if you want to be healthy and prevent disease! So why not love yourself to the max by cutting out the red and going green?

In addition to halting the accumulation of plaque, a proper plant-based diet can also reverse the process entirely. In a groundbreaking study, Dr. Dean Ornish of the Preventative Medicine Research Institute in California assembled 48 patients suffering from severe heart disease. Twenty participants continued their typical animal-based Western diet, while the other 28 adopted a strict, plant-based regimen along with performing basic stretching and walking exercises.

The results? A staggering 82 percent of the participants in the plant-based group witnessed a reduction in their arterial blockage. And in one dramatic case, Werner Hebenstreit, a seventy-five-year-old businessman, had improved so much he was able to hike at over 8,000 feet for six hours in the Grand Tetons. Before beginning a plant-based diet, he could barely cross the street without experiencing chest pains.

Meanwhile, of those meat munchers who continued with the typical

Western diet, none got better, and in most cases their arterial blockage continued to worsen.

Still skeptical? Consider the story of a guy named Bill. Bill grew up in the South eating a traditional animal-based diet, and was partial to fried chicken, hamburgers, and French fries. He was even known for ducking into McDonald's during his weekly jogs. But years of red meat and fried foods took their toll, and in 2004, Bill underwent quadruple coronary-artery bypass surgery.

In 2010, doctors had to insert stents into his native coronary after one of those bypasses failed. (The frequency of bypass procedures failing within one-and-a-half years is quite high, according to a 2009 article in the *New England Journal of Medicine*. Almost 50 percent of the time, the vessel taken from your leg and used to bypass your blocked artery will shut down within twelve to eighteen months.)

Bill's daughter was upset and soon demanded that her father improve his health before her wedding later that year. So Bill started poring over the peer-reviewed scientific literature and, inspired by my father's twenty-five years of research reversing heart disease in hundreds of patients at the Cleveland Clinic, as well as the work of Dr. Dean Ornish and T. Colin Campbell, dove into the plant-strong sea of goodness and changed his diet! Bill ultimately dropped twenty-five pounds, and walked his daughter down the aisle not long afterward.

You may have heard of Bill. He was the forty-second president of the United States. So take it from President Clinton, who recently told an interviewer, "I live on a plant-based diet of beans, legumes, vegetables, and fruit...I want to be one of the 82 percent of people who reverse their heart disease."

2

Plants Are Plentiful in Protein

A few years ago, when I was still a firefighter, we were on an assistance call to lift a 600-pound woman out of her room and into a waiting ambulance. When we arrived at her bedroom, we found it littered with pizza boxes, empty buckets of fried chicken, and dozens of drained soda bottles—all the evidence we needed to know why she was morbidly obese. As the eight of us were grunting, groaning, and struggling to lift her, I nicely suggested that she might consider eating less refined food and more fresh, whole plants. She looked up at me, baffled, and asked, "But where would I get my protein?"

Meat eaters throw a lot of false facts at you, but maybe the most common one is this: You can't get enough protein eating plants.

Puh-leeeeeeeez! Stop the nonsense!! There is *no* such thing as protein deficiency in the United States. How many people do you know who were hospitalized last year for protein deficiency? Zero! Now, how many people do you know who were hospitalized for heart disease, cancer, diabetes, or obesity-related ailments? Probably lots.

In fact, the majority of Americans are walking around in a state of protein *overload*—and it's little wonder. We live in a country that is head over heels in love with anything that even smells of protein. We've been so hoodwinked and bamboozled by the meat, milk, and egg industries that the majority of people, including well-meaning but misinformed doctors and nutritionists, haven't a clue that the best and most healthful sources of protein come from whole plants.

Yes, plants! So take a seat, because we're about to get real about protein. Let me start by giving you an analogy. If you are breathing air, you're probably pretty confident you're getting enough oxygen. Air is 21 percent oxygen and 79 percent nitrogen—but you're not overly worried about getting enough oxygen. As long as your lungs are taking in air, you're a happy camper and figure you're in good shape.

Now think about food and protein. If you're eating food, it doesn't really matter which foods you're eating—as long as you're taking in enough calories, you can pretty much rest assured you're also getting enough protein. Yes, protein is of prime importance, and is the most plentiful substance in the body besides water—but that doesn't mean eating more of it is better for you.

Many authorities, including the World Health Organization, recommend that protein should make up at least 10 percent of total calories in the human diet. The crazy thing is that most of us are getting much more than we need in terms of protein and calories.

In addition, because most Americans eat so much meat and so few whole, plant-based foods, most of the protein our body has to work with is coming from an unfriendly source, namely animal protein. And animal protein is bad for our bones, creates an inflammatory state in our bodies, increases the risk of tumor development, raises cholesterol levels, and is harsh on the liver and kidneys.

For healthy individuals, the World Health Organization recommends the following formula to calculate your daily protein requirements: (0.8 grams) × (your ideal body weight in kilograms) = protein in grams. So, for a 175-pound guy like me using the above formula I should be getting 64 grams of protein per day. This is an absolute snap!

So instead of relying on a third-class version of protein, why not go to the mother source—healthful and healing plants. Let's look at the amount of protein found in plant-based foods, so you can feel confident you're getting all the protein you need from eating them.

Twenty-five percent of the calories in your average vegetable come from protein—with many leafy green vegetables boasting as much as 50 percent! Your average bean contains 25 percent protein—soybeans as much as 40 percent. Your average whole grain contains 12 percent protein—quinoa as much as 18 percent. And even your average fruit contains well over 5 percent protein—lemons as much as 15 percent. So take those lemons and make lemonade!

Here is a list of several fruits and their protein content, according to the U.S. Department of Agriculture (USDA) food database:

Oranges (1 navel): 7.4 percent
Strawberries (1 cup, whole): 8.3 percent
Kiwi (1 whole fruit or 1 cup, sliced): 7.5 percent
Apple (1 medium): 2 percent
Pineapple (1 cup, chunks): 4.3 percent
Peaches (1 medium): 9.3 percent
Banana (1 medium): 4.9 percent

As you can see, theoretically you could almost be a fruitarian in Fiji and still not run the risk of being protein deficient (not recommended, however!).

In fact, protein deficiency is so rare that I have never found a *single* person who knows the name of the medical condition that results from a serious lack of it in the diet. Not one person. What is that word? The answer is on page 18.

The only two ways to blow it with protein are by (1) not consuming enough calories to maintain a healthy weight, and (2) eating mostly foods that are high in fat and sugar (the chips, donuts, French-fries-and-soda-pop diet). If you're eating an unprocessed plant-strong diet while keeping a healthy weight, you're covered!

A Protein Flash About Flesh

We all know that without protein, we can't survive. But nature is pretty smart, and has designed humans in a way that ensures our survival even with little protein from food. Why? Because of a process called "protein turnover" that takes place in our body. According to the classic textbook *Nutrition* (Insel, Ross, fourth edition, 2012), cells throughout the body constantly synthesize and break down protein, leaving behind amino acids, some of which are then used for protein synthesis. Of the approximately 300 grams of protein synthesized by the body each day, 200 grams come from these recycled amino acids. This cycle takes place every day of your life, without your having to do a thing. So the next time someone asks you where you get most of your protein from, just tell them from human flesh!

3

Plant-Based Proteins Are Completely Complete

The second big and widespread misconception about protein is that plant proteins are somehow not "complete."

This one's not only not factual, it's not even a smart opinion. It is a fallacy, based on outdated research that was weak to begin with. So when someone slips this myth into conversation, take a deep breath and set up for an overhead slam.

But first, let's look at the definition of proteins. Proteins are nutrients made up of one or more chains of amino acids, which are essential to the structure, function, and regulation of every cell in your body. In fact, proteins are the most plentiful substance in the human body besides water.

The nomenclature surrounding proteins is the first source of misinformation about them. Each protein chain contains twenty amino acids, eight of which (called "essential amino acids") can be obtained only through food. Foods with all eight essential amino acids are known as "complete" proteins. These foods include various types of meat, poultry, fish, eggs, milk, dairy, fruits, vegetables, whole grains, beans, nuts, and seeds. Yes, you heard me: fruits, vegetables, whole grains, beans, nuts, and seeds! The foods that you might sometimes hear called "incomplete" proteins aren't incomplete at all! In fact, the only incomplete protein in food comes from an animal-based source: gelatin.

Some people believe that they have to combine different plant-based foods to create "complete" proteins. This belief, called "protein combining," was a theory initially put forward in the 1971 bestseller *Diet for a Small Planet* by Frances Moore Lappé. It quickly became one of the biggest myths in the dieting world. Ten years later, Lappé herself formally rescinded her position in a new edition of the same book: "In combating the myth that meat is the only way to get high-quality protein, I reinforced another myth. I gave the impression that in order to get enough protein without meat, considerable care was needed in choosing foods. Actually, it is much easier than I thought."

By then, the damage had been done, but influential food-related organizations eventually began to come around. In 1988, for example, the Academy of Nutrition and Dietetics also amended its position on plant-based proteins. The organization's most recent statement on vegetarianism galvanizes their previous support of plant proteins:

"Plant protein can meet protein requirements when a variety of plant foods is consumed and energy needs are met. Research indicates that an assortment of plant foods eaten over the course of a day can provide all essential amino acids and ensure adequate nitrogen retention and use in healthy adults; thus, complementary proteins do not need to be consumed at the same meal."

Translation: Don't sweat it! You can eat a plant-strong diet and get your protein groove on.

So here's the deal: Animal proteins and plant proteins are both complete. The difference is that the composition and proportion of the amino acids in animal protein are higher in the sulfur-containing amino acids, which in excess may be harmful.

On the flip side, plant proteins have a healthier composition and balance of essential amino acids, one that has been elegantly balanced by nature in a way that inherently protects us from inflammation and tumor growth. In addition, plants come with added gifts such as fiber, phytonutrients, and antioxidants. All of which are sorely missing in meat.

So the next time someone questions you on the dangers of eating a plant-based diet that is "lacking" or "incomplete" in protein, let that person know you have found the mother source of protein, and it's spelled P.L.A.N.T.S.!!

How Would You Prefer to Get Your Protein?

I trust you'll agree that most balanced diets, including plant-based ones, contain more than enough protein, and that protein deficiency is utterly a nonissue for anyone living in the United States. What is an issue is the package your protein comes in.

This is where we herbivores really outstrip our carnivorous cousins—ounce for ounce, beans may have less protein than bacon, but they are so much better for us.

For example, let's look at a 6-ounce, broiled porterhouse steak. It contains lots of clunky animal protein (38 grams), but is also chock-full of saturated fat (16 grams). In comparison, 1 cup of cooked lentils has 18 grams of classy plant protein and less than 1 gram of total fat—and zero saturated fat.

The best protein packages for the health conscious are found in lean, friendly, nutritious, fiber-filled plants such as beans, peas, lentils, green leafy vegetables, whole grains, and nuts and soy products, including tofu, tempeh, and edamame.

(The name of the disease caused by insufficient dietary protein is *kwashiorkor*. How many times have you heard that word?)

4

Vitamin B12:
Not a Problem!

I'm willing to bet that another argument you'll hear all the time is: If you don't eat meat, you'll die from lack of vitamin B12!

What most misinformed meat eaters don't know is that vitamin B12 doesn't originate in animals—or plants, for that matter. Vitamin B12 is actually found in soil and is made from microorganisms that live in our environment. But before you decide to dive into a pile of dirt and start chomping away, let's take a look at vitamin B12's history.

B12 was the last vitamin to be discovered (in 1948), and only accidentally, while scientists were searching for a cure for a disease called pernicious anemia (a terrible condition that stops the body from making enough red blood cells). It turns out vitamin B12 cures it, along with many other disorders. So everyone needs B12.

Now, most people know that they can get vitamin B12 from eating meat—and meat eaters love to tell you this. But here's what they probably don't know (and what you should feel free to inform them): It's actually not the meat itself that gives animals their B12. It comes from the plants the animals eat, and specifically from the dirt that is attached to the plants!

So where should you get your vitamin B12 if you set sail on the plant-strong course for years to come?

You could eat more dirt, and actually, if you live near an organic farm that sells fresh vegetables with a little dirt on them, that's not a bad idea. However, for most of us, the answer is B12 supplementation. Take a pill (either 100 to 200 micrograms [mcg] once a day, or two 1000-mcg pills twice a week. If pills aren't your thing, say hello to fortified whole-grain cereals, the smorgasbord of plant-based milks at your disposal, and/or various brands of nutritional yeast that contain B12.

How much B12 is necessary? The RDA for vitamin B12 is a min-uscule 2.4 mcg. A plant-based eater can get that much at breakfast from fortified cereal, which contains anywhere from 1.5 to 6 mcg per cup, depending on the brand. Soy-based "meats" contain 2 mcg to 7 mcg, and fortified plant milks can range from 0.2 mcg to 5 mcg per serving.

And by the way, even if you forget to take your vitamin B12 one morning, all week, or even all month, there's no need to start freaking out. Humans have, on average, a staggering three- to five-year supply of B12 stored in the liver.

If you don't know your B12 level, it's not a bad idea to have your doctor test it. I do this, and mine is 854. A normal blood level is 250 to 1100 picograms per milliliter.

B12 and Seniors

Here's something I learned from Brenda Davis, a fantastic nutritional consultant and author of the excellent book *Becoming Vegan*.

Brenda explains that, in all animal products, vitamin B12 is bound to protein. So, to absorb that B12 from these products, we must cleave the B12 off of the protein to which it is bound. For most people this doesn't seem to be a problem, but between 10 and 30 percent of people aged fifty-plus cannot do this (or at least, not very well).

The reason is that to separate the B12 off of the protein, our body needs to produce sufficient enzymes and stomach acid. We tend to lose both of these as we age. This is why the U.S. Food and Nutrition Board recommends that everyone older than fifty years rely on B12-fortified foods or supplements rather than animal products for B12.

5

Plants Are Iron-Strong

There's a reason why the most grueling triathlon competition is called the "IronMan." Iron has long symbolized strength and power. And it's absolutely essential to life. Iron supplies oxygen to blood and muscles, assists biochemical reactions, helps in cell growth, and is essential for good health. Without it, you'll come down with fatigue, compromised immune response, headaches, heart murmurs, and more.

Many of the meat eaters lurking out there will pop out from behind a hanging cow carcass (like the one Rocky Balboa slugged into mincemeat) and tell you the only way to get iron is from meat. But your susceptibility to iron deficiency doesn't depend on whether or not you eat meat. In fact, iron deficiency affects Americans on all diets; studies comparing vegetarians and vegans to omnivores have shown no correlation between diet and iron deficiency.

So, yes, we all want to be iron men and women. And figuring out how much iron we need and the best way to get it doesn't have to be like a high school physics experiment.

Iron deficiency is actually the most common nutritional deficiency in the world. The World Health Organization (WHO) estimates that two billion people, or more than 30 percent of the world's population, are anemic, often due to iron deficiency. Furthermore, lack of iron is one of only a few nutritional deficiencies found in industrialized countries like the United States where, WHO says, it "exacts its heaviest overall toll in terms of ill-health, premature death, and lost earnings."

There are two types of dietary iron: heme and non-heme. Heme iron comes from hemoglobin, and can only be obtained by eating animals that once had red blood cells. Foods with heme iron include red meats, poultry, and fish. The iron derived from plants, which don't bleed, is non-heme. This is also the type of iron used to fortify foods.

Some uninformed sorts will tell you that meat is a better source of iron than plants because heme iron is absorbed more efficiently by the body, at rates ranging from 15 percent to 35 percent. In contrast, non-heme iron is absorbed at rates ranging from 2 percent to 20 percent. Non-heme iron absorption is also influenced by other foods eaten with it. For example, vitamin C will greatly boost absorption by about 30 percent; dairy products and the oxalates in certain leafy greens blunt absorption.

Before this starts sounding like an argument for meat eating, I'll tell you a secret: You don't need as much iron as you think. According to the CDC, a man like me (between 19 and 50 years old) needs 8 milligrams (mg) of iron per day. However, since I don't eat meat, and I will be absorbing less of the non-heme iron entering my body, that number rises slightly to 14 mg.

Seem like a lot? Nope. A cup of soybeans contains 8.8 mg, a cup of lentils 6.6 mg, and a tablespoon of blackstrap molasses 3.5 mg. (Remember, you can also boost the amount you absorb of these numbers by 30 percent if you are consuming some form of vitamin C with your meal.)

In addition, cooking in an iron skillet increases the iron content in many foods. For example, the Academy of Nutrition and Dietetics found that the iron in 100 grams of spaghetti sauce rocketed from 0.6 mg to 5.7 mg after being cooked in a cast-iron pot.

Women and children need to be more vigilant about their iron intake than men. On the high end, it's recommended that pregnant women on plant-based diets eat about 30 milligrams of iron a day to compensate for their babies. Women also lose iron during their monthly menstrual periods, but how much varies according to how light or heavy the periods are. Besides women and children, those who need to consume higher levels of iron include adolescents, athletes (especially endurance athletes), and the elderly. Consulting with a nutritionist is always a helpful way to determine how much iron you should have in your diet.

When you're computing how to get that iron, one of the biggest advantages of non-heme iron from plants is that it comes without the calorie count. For instance, a cup of cooked spinach offers 6.4 mg of iron at only 6.6 calories. One serving (3 ounces) of beef tenderloin offers 3 mg of iron and 247 calories. Which would you rather eat?

By the way, excess iron in the body is not a good thing. It is associated with the formation of free radicals, those nasty little atoms that cause degenerative diseases, heart disease, and cancer. High consumption of heme iron also raises the risk of gallstones in men. Some scientists advise that people with diets rich in heme iron offset it by consuming foods that blunt iron absorption, such as dairy products and tannins (found in tea).

If you are wondering what the best sources of non-heme iron are, the following table from the U.S. government's fact sheet on iron will get you started:

Food	Milligrams per serving	% Daily Value*
Ready-to-eat cereal, 100% iron fortified, ¾ cup	18.0	100
Oatmeal, instant, fortified, prepared with water, 1 cup	10.0	60
Soybeans, mature, boiled, 1 cup	8.8	50
Lentils, boiled, 1 cup	6.6	35
Beans, kidney, mature, boiled, 1 cup	5.2	25
Beans, lima, large, mature, boiled, 1 cup	4.5	25
Beans, navy, mature, boiled, 1 cup	4.5	25
Ready-to-eat cereal, 25% iron fortified, ¾ cup	4.5	25
Beans, black, mature, boiled, 1 cup	3.6	20
Beans, pinto, mature, boiled, 1 cup	3.6	20
Molasses, blackstrap, 1 tablespoon	3.5	20
Tofu, raw, firm, ½ cup	3.4	20
Spinach, boiled, drained, ½ cup	3.2	20

Finally, if you want to complement your iron intake with vitamin C in order to boost absorption, try some of these tasty options along with your iron-clad meal: red bell pepper, green bell pepper, Brussels sprouts, broccoli, sweet potato, kale, kiwi, orange, mango, and/or grapefruit.

Bottom line: Heme iron from meat is an inferior, unregulated locomotive going all over the place and getting you nowhere. However, plant-indigenous iron is a superior, regulated city bus that obeys all the traffic signs and drops everyone off at their proper destination.

6

Plants Are Bone-Strong

Whenever I give a presentation and it's time to talk about calcium, the first thing I ask the audience is, "Who can tell me where calcium comes from?" A handful of people always jump up and excitedly call out "A cow!"

Come on, people! Calcium does not originate with a cow. It's not "cow-cium"! It's calcium. Calcium is a mineral, and minerals come from the soil. Therefore, the best place to get your calcium is from the best conduit of calcium—plants. With plants you are getting a superior form of calcium that is highly absorbable because of the alkaline (non-acidic) and friendly nature of the leafy greens, beans, and seeds that are an efficient transport system for plant-retainable calcium that will *really* help you build strong bones and a strong body. A body built by plants, not cow secretions!

Really? No cow's milk? But what about all the warnings? "Drink lots of milk or else your bones will get old and frail and crumble before your first social security check arrives in the mail."

Thanks to those Got Milk? ads, along with armies of dairy industry lobbyists, most people are taught to believe that because dairy products do contain calcium, we should, therefore, guzzle milk by the gallon, in between trays full of cheese plates (or cottage cheese, for the diet-conscious).

And doesn't Big Milk have a lot of credibility with experts? After all, the Surgeon General, the CDC, the National Institutes of Health, and the National Osteoporosis Foundation all have gone on record to say that milk is what keeps our bones from crumbling.

I say, question authority. Question it when the former head of the American Heart Association, Clyde Yancy, states: "This kind [of heart] disease is progressive. There aren't any cures." And yet the peer-reviewed scientific literature says something entirely different. Question it when President Clinton's cardiologist, Allan Schwartz, asserts: "This is not a result of his [Bill's] lifestyle or diet. This is a chronic condition. We don't have a cure for this condition." And yet the former fast-food president himself has flipped to plants, and regained his health, because the evidence over the last twenty-five years supporting a low-fat, plant-based diet is so overwhelming.

It's the same with these big organizations backing dairy. As it turns out, the science behind many of Big Milk's claims is crumbling. According to recent studies, more than one-half of postmenopausal women in America now have either osteopenia (reduced bone mass that may be a prelude to osteoporosis) or osteoporosis (literally, "porous bones"). Osteoporosis is called the "silent disease" because there are often no symptoms until the bones begin to fail and break.

Or look at some relevant data from two very different peoples: black South Africans and Canadian Inuits. If dairy consumption prevents osteoporosis, the South Africans, who consume little dairy, should have epidemic levels of the disease. Actually, the reverse is true: The prevalence of osteoporosis-related diseases in black South Africans is among the lowest in the world. On the other hand, the Inuit have the highest dietary calcium intake of any people in the world, and they also show the highest osteoporosis rates in the world.

The countries that consume the most dairy products—those in Northern Europe along with the United States, New Zealand, and Australia—actually have the highest bone fracture rates. In fact, regions that consume the lowest amounts of dairy—eastern Asia and Africa—boast fracture rates 50 to 70 percent lower than we milk guzzlers.

So what gives? The truth is while calcium certainly helps our bones stay strong, we only need moderate amounts of it. Since 1975, there have been nearly 140 clinical trials studying the link between dairy consumption and bone density, and two-thirds of them found that dairy-intensive diets did not promote stronger bones. In fact, the Harvard Nurses' Study, an investigation into osteoporosis and bone loss in women, showed that "Fracture rates were higher for those who consumed three or more servings, compared to those who did not drink milk."

Think of it this way. Peanut butter cups contain small amounts of vitamin K, but I challenge you to find a doctor who'd recommend eating 150 peanut butter cups a day for your daily vitamin K intake. While you might get your vitamin K, all that fat and sugar will destroy your body faster than you can say Willy Wonka.

The same goes for calcium. Remember that dairy and meat products contain a lot of animal protein, which itself is chock-full of amino acids that cascade through our bloodstream. In order to neutralize these acids, the body needs to release something alkaline to restore our natural pH balance. And guess what? One of the most effective alkalizing agents is the calcium stored in our bones. So while that chocolate milk you're drinking might have a lot of calcium, its high animal-protein content ironically ends up siphoning essential calcium from your bones! Holy osteoporosis, Batman!

Our sources of calcium become increasingly important with age. Younger bodies are actively building and rebuilding bones to make them stronger; that's why kids heal so fast after breaking something. In fact, until the age of about thirty, our bodies consistently build more bone than is lost. After that, our bones slowly weaken and lose their elasticity.

So if you want to have strong bones and be healthy, here's the trick! Avoid diets rich in animal-based proteins, which will decrease the pH level of our blood, draining that precious calcium from our bones. And although your milk-guzzling friends may seem healthy now, that may not be the case in a few decades.

Don't believe it? Consider this: There is more calcium in 4 ounces of the average serving of (calcium fortified) firm tofu—or in ¾ cup of collard greens—than a whole glass of milk! And if you find yourself still craving a milky treat, try chocolate soy milk. Most soy milk is fortified with more calcium than cow's milk, and because it doesn't contain any of those nasty animal proteins, your blood's pH level stays nice and stable.

And despite their humble appearance, good old beans are some of the most robust, bone-buildin' grub around. Just 2 cups of black beans contains more than 90 mg of calcium, and a cup of delicious white beans has a whopping 130 mg. Other great veggie sources of calcium include soybeans, bok choy, broccoli, collard greens, kale, and sweet potatoes.

Instead of Got Milk?, it should be Got Saturated Fat? Think of milk as liquid meat. Did you know that an 8-ounce glass of whole milk has the same amount of saturated fat as 4.5 slices of bacon and four times the calories? An 8-ounce glass of 2-percent-fat milk has the same amount of saturated fat as 3 slices of bacon and the same amount of calories. And an 8-ounce glass of 1-percent milk has more saturated fat than a strip of bacon, more than twice the calories, and 35 percent more cholesterol. That's not doing any body any good!

*   *   *

Your milk-guzzling friends still think you're nuts? Maybe they're onto something. As it happens, some nuts are a great source of calcium. A handful of almonds is packed with 75 mg of calcium, along with plenty of protein and fiber. And just three Brazil nuts pack in about 22 mg of calcium.

So remember, all calcium sources aren't created equal. Your bones need the premium fuel, and a plant-based diet packs the purest, highest-octane stuff around.

Keep in mind: If you take this data to heart and avoid milk, be prepared, because when you tell your family and friends that you're no longer drinking it, they will look at you as if you were an unpatriotic turncoat. This is to be expected, because we've been so indoctrinated into believing that milk and milk by-products are the perfect foods to build a strong body and bones that anyone questioning it seems treasonous.

But think about it. How many people in your life do you know who are guzzling milk, choking down cheese, and gobbling up Greek yogurt every day of the week? I bet lots and lots! And yet we have an epidemic of osteoporosis in this country. Something does not compute. Americans are consuming dairy in quantities far greater than even the dairy industry's marketing plea for three servings daily, and yet dairy is doing nothing to protect our bones.

In addition to eating a plant-strong diet, the best ways to guarantee strong bones are to limit sodium intake, ditch the soft drinks, quit smoking, curb the dairy, and engage in weight-bearing exercise two to three times a week. Here come some strong bones!

Harvard Hates Milk

Just as 2011 turned into 2012, Harvard University turned into a strong force against dairy. In response to the United States Department of Agriculture's (USDA) new MyPlate guide for healthy eating, the Harvard School of Public Health released its own "Healthy Eating Plate" food guide. Unlike the USDA's, Harvard's food guide was not influenced by food industry lobbyists! It's as pure as it gets. And what did it say about dairy? "High intake can increase the risk of prostate cancer and possibly ovarian cancer." Instead, it recommended you get your calcium from foods such as dark leafy greens, collards, fortified soy milk, and baked beans. Go Crimson!

7

Humans Are Herbivores

How many times have you heard this one: "Our ancestors ate meat, so why should we limit ourselves to only plants?"

Or how about this one: "If we weren't meant to eat meat, why have people been doing it for so many thousands of years?"

These arguments are not technically lies, but they're hardly the full story, either. Some of our ancestors did eat meat, but that's only part of a much more complex story that includes thousands of years of human cultural and biological evolution. The truth is: Just because we *can* eat meat doesn't mean that we *should*.

For early humans, meat was a concentrated package of calories and nutrients that fueled their incredibly labor-intensive lifestyles at a time when food scarcity was common. As my friend and nutrition expert Dr. John McDougall writes: "A traditional Arctic Eskimo, living in a subfreezing climate, could expend 6,000 calories and more a day just to keep warm and hunt for food. The high-fat animal food sources—fish, walrus, whale, and seal—from his local environment were the most practical means of meeting the demands of those rigorous surroundings."

However, modern life, with its office jobs, cars, and central heating, does not exactly impose the same physical demands on the human body. For this reason, those concentrated packages of calories and nutrients don't make sense, says Dr. McDougall. "Modern Eskimos living in heated houses and driving around in their climate-controlled SUVs, still consuming a high-meat diet, have become some of the fattest and sickest people on earth."

If we no longer need to eat meat, then why have our bodies evolved to eat it? The truth is that they haven't in an efficient and healthy way, and that's because our physiology has much more in common with herbivores than with carnivores.

Let's take a tour with Dr. Milton Mills, an expert in the anatomy of herbivores vs. carnivores.

Start with the mouth: Carnivores' mouths consist of a jaw with a simple hinge joint and relatively little musculature. They have short, pointed incisors, elongated canines for cutting and tearing flesh, and triangular, jagged-edged molars that work like serrated knives. Their saliva contains no digestive juices.

The saliva of herbivores, in comparison, is full of an enzyme called alpha-amylase that helps digest the complex carbohydrates found in plants. Carnivores don't need this enzyme because meat doesn't contain carbohydrates. Their mouths are made to cut and tear large hunks of flesh from the bone and then swallow it whole, without mastication.

Human mouths exhibit the same characteristics as those of herbivores. We have large, well-developed lips, and muscular jaws that can move side to side and back and forth to aid in biting off and mashing up plant matter. We also have spade-like incisors and square, flattened molars, better for grinding and chewing than chomping and sheering. Even our canines are comparatively blunt compared with the dagger-like teeth of carnivores.

And our saliva? Chock-full of alpha-amylase.

Heading down into a carnivore's stomach, in the belly of the beast you find a large (compared to its body size) stomach, a bubbling cauldron of highly concentrated acid followed by a short, straight, and relatively simple intestine. The stomach needs to be large because meat eaters eat relatively infrequently, and when they do they need to be able to gorge themselves all at once, then digest later. The highly acidic stomach juices are necessary to dissolve the large quantity of muscle and bone materials that carnivores swallow, and to kill the bacteria in the rotting meat that could otherwise kill the animal. The intestines are designed to move food quickly out of the system so that it does not begin to putrefy.

The human stomach, again like that of other herbivores, is smaller and only moderately acidic because digesting fruits, vegetables, and grains is much less of a labor-intensive task. Our intestines are long and coiled, slowing the digestion process and allowing our bodies to break down foods slowly and to absorb more nutrients from them. Crucially, our large intestines have a pouched structure that is only seen elsewhere in the large intestines of herbivores.

As food digests, the liver clears some of its more harmful elements from the body. The liver of a carnivore rids its body of 100 percent of the cholesterol that enters it through eating meat (remember, kooky cholesterol only exists in meat). Our human livers, on the other hand, are very bad at getting rid of the stuff, a problem that causes cholesterol to build up in our arteries (a process called atherosclerosis) and results in heart attacks.

Another curious feature of our digestive system is its need for certain vitamins. Animals have a tendency to evolve in relationship to available foods. Carnivores, who were unable to get ascorbic acid, or vitamin C, from their diets (as it is found only in plants), instead evolved to synthesize it in their own bodies.

Humans, who have always eaten plants, have no such ability and depend on their diets to get vitamin C.

So eating meat isn't a biological necessity. But why did our ancestors do it? Although some people might want to view them all as happy, club-wielding cave dwellers who feasted on mastodons and wooly mammoths, the truth is that their diets varied greatly depending on the periods during which they lived. The earliest humans probably ate an almost exclusively plant-based diet, while further down the timeline they turned to hunting and gathering, which effectively flipped their diet into one that included meat.

Then, with the advent of farming roughly 10,000 years ago, our fickle ancestors flopped back to mostly plant-based eating, a trend that can be seen as recently as the era of feudal Japan. So history shows us that more than being meat eaters, humans have always been opportunistic eaters who are much more likely to follow environmental trends than what biology actually dictates.

Best-selling writer and zoologist Desmond Morris has written extensively about human dietary preferences. In his book *The Naked Ape*, he discusses why, despite our meat-eating habits, humans are better suited for plant eating. "It could be argued that, since our primate ancestors had to make do without a major meat component in their diets, we should be able to do the same," he writes. "We were driven to become flesh-eaters only by environmental circumstances, and now that we have the environment under control, with elaborately cultivated crops at our disposal, we might be expected to return to our ancient primate feeding patterns."

Meat eating may well have played an important part in our human past. In hunter-gatherer societies, where bringing home the bison was a full-time job, meat was a calorie-packed supplement to an otherwise plant-based diet. But in the twenty-first century, most of us have full-time jobs where failure doesn't imply starvation. We are trying to take calories *out* of our diets, not pack them in. Food is readily available in the most benign hunting ground imaginable—the supermarket.

If meat was a necessity for us at various moments in our natural history, we've long since evolved past it. Yet some people insist on living in the past—particularly the Paleo dieters. (For more on the Paleo people, see chapter 11.)

8

The Many Myths of Meat

Meat is a must." "Meat, it's what's for dinner." "Humans can't live without meat."

Do you ever wonder where we get all this good news about meat?

Try the meat industry itself. The U.S. cattle industry alone had $74 billion in sales in 2010 (for 26.4 billion pounds of beef) and you can bet your rump steak that a hefty chunk of that went into political lobbying. The sad truth is that the information we get about health often has more to do with politics and money than with science and fact. Meat eaters are misinformed for good reason. Most companies involved in the meat business are represented by one of three lobbying groups: the American Meat Institute, the National Meat Association, and the National Cattlemen's Beef Association. Their influence goes right to the top.

When Michael Taylor was appointed by the Clinton Administration as head of the Food Safety and Inspection Service (the meat watchdog branch of the USDA), two names already present on the speed-dial of his office phone were the American Meat Institute and the National Cattlemen's Beef Association. The USDA has been in cahoots with these guys since its inception in 1862, because it has always had the dual mandate of protecting American agricultural interests *and* advising the public about food choices. In plain speak, this is called "the fox guarding the henhouse." Or as my father likes to say, "This would be like having Al Capone do your taxes."

The classic example of the USDA's conflicting roles came when the creation of the food pyramid in 1991 was delayed for a year and a day because of pressure from the meat industry. Just days before the pyramid was set to debut, Marian Burros of the *New York Times* broke the news that the Washington-based health advocacy group Physicians Committee for Responsible Medicine (PCRM) had asked the USDA to make its four food groups completely plant based: fruits, vegetables, whole grains, and legumes—and the carnivores had a cow!

Even though the USDA declined the request, the Cattlemen's Association called an emergency meeting with the Secretary of Agriculture, Richard Madigan (who had just attained the position with the support of commodity and farm groups). The trade groups complained that the proposed pyramid would hurt meat consumption. In response to the complaint, the USDA spent another $855,000 on research in order to confirm what they already knew—that you should eat more of every other food but meat.

If you think that sounds bad, try this: In 1995, the meat industry did everything it could to stop the USDA from implementing food-safety regulations that would require testing for salmonella in ground beef. The stampede was led by Representative James Walsh (who received $65,000 from agriculture-industry companies during the 1996 election). And although Walsh was unable to stop the rules from being implemented, the cattle industry went on to challenge the USDA in the Supreme Court, and won. Based on that decision, the USDA still can't shut down a ground beef plant based solely on salmonella levels in the beef.

Hold on to your cowboy hats, because the meat lobbyists look like wimps compared with the Center for Consumer Freedom (CCF). The tobacco lobbyist Rick Berman founded this group with nearly $3 million from Philip Morris, back before they changed their name to Altria Group to distance themselves from the fact that their products, including cigarettes, were deadly to their own customers.

The Center is dedicated to "shooting the messenger," Berman-speak for discrediting any groups that try to publicize the health risks of the products produced by the companies that pay them, namely tobacco, junk food, and, you guessed it, meat. The Center for Consumer Freedom and its buddy the American Meat Institute have been trying to smear PCRM (our friends who recommended that the four main food groups be plant based) for years.

Other recent CCF campaigns have targeted the WHO, because it addressed obesity; the CDC, for investigating food safety; and even Mothers Against Drunk Driving, for some reason.

Our steak-and-kidney-pie-eating friends across the pond are playing the same game. A high-profile study released in 2011 by the British Nutrition Foundation concluded that people *shouldn't* reduce their meat intake—but there wouldn't have been a study if the British meat industry hadn't funded it.

Besides dissing plant eating, the meat industry is constantly thinking up ways to make its product seem healthier. Get a load of this: There is an online, six-hour college course offered by the National Cattlemen's Beef Association called The Masters of Beef Advocacy. Yep. It's available in forty-seven states. Students who receive their so-called MBA are then expected to speak at schools or promote meat through social media.

If such advocacy fails, the industry may personally go after anyone who threatens their message. This includes schools. In 2009, Baltimore city schools implemented a "Meatless Monday" program in their cafeterias as a way for the chronically short-funded school system to save money and fight rising obesity rates among students. When the American Meat Institute got wind of it, they went straight to CNN to complain that American children weren't getting enough protein. Then, as the "Meatless Monday" movement gained steam with celebrity chefs like Mario Batali, the meat lobbyists went into overdrive, sending threatening letters to organizations that had adopted the movement and campaigning against it on the Internet.

The good news is that even the powers that be are slowly coming around to the sad realities about meat. They are reading the studies and reviewing the research. The USDA's latest plant-strong, plate-shaped food guide of fruits, vegetables, whole grains, and protein has eliminated the "meat" group entirely and replaced it with "protein," showing that you don't need to eat meat to have a healthful and balanced diet. Ever. So don't think you do. Don't buy the "B.S." I certainly don't, and haven't since 1987.

The Beef Council Meets Engine 2

A few months after *The Engine 2 Diet* hit the shelves in February of 2009, all forty-four Austin fire stations got a visit from a representative of the Texas Beef Council, delivering a fully cooked warm brisket, plus grilling tools, an "ultimate grilling guide," an apron, and a letter. In the letter, the Council mentioned that "in light of *The Engine 2 Diet*, we wanted to provide you, as key influencers of the community, with these gifts to honor you for all you do." This certainly got people talking, and although many of the guys gobbled up the free brisket, I got many more phone calls from fellow firefighters letting me know that I should write more books so the stations could get more free stuff.

The reality is the meat eaters at the trade associations didn't like Engine 2 muscling in on their territory. Tough. They should feel threatened, because the tides they are a-turning!

9

Grass-Fed Beef Is No Better Than Grain-Fed

Sometimes, when you're in the middle of an argument with meat eaters, they'll throw this one at you: We don't eat any old meat. We eat meat from *grass-fed* cows, which are healthier, safer, and more environmentally friendly than regular cows.

Yeah, it sounds good. "Grass fed." But in reality, there isn't much difference between grass-fed and regular grain-fed cows. For starters, most cows are raised outside eating grasses for the first two-thirds of their lives, so there's nothing special about that. Regular beef cows then spend the last third of their lives eating a mix of corn and other grains spiked with hormones and growth supplements. If you think this means that grass feeding is more humane, think again. Grass-fed cows can still be put in feedlots and pumped full of hormones just like any other cow, but as long as they don't eat any grains they maintain their special status.

Given their similar breeding, it's no surprise that the two types of meat aren't very different either, diet-wise. If the average American switched all of his/her meat consumption from grain-fed to grass-fed meat, he/she would save just 16,642 calories a year—that's about eight days' worth of calories.

You aren't helping the environment, either. Cows that spend their lives grazing in a pasture aren't good for the environment; they are just less bad than cows that spend their lives in holding pens. A diet of natural grasses cuts down on the resource cost of production, but maintains the same amounts of soil erosion, manure runoff, and especially methane gas emissions. Raising cattle—grass fed or otherwise—ranks among the leading causes of global warming. Although they may consume negligibly fewer resources than their factory-farm brethren, grass-fed livestock still contribute massive amounts of CO_2. According to the United Nations, livestock account for 9 percent of all CO_2 emissions—more than all cars and trucks and planes combined! Moreover, livestock contribute a disproportionately large share of nitrous oxide, which has 296 times the Global Warming Potential (GWP) as CO_2. Most emissions are a result of manure, which is a stinky inevitability no matter how much grass you feed a cow.

Another grass-fed myth is that these animals are far happier than they would be on a conventional factory farm. Grass-fed cows are still forcibly impregnated, an extremely painful and inhumane procedure. Infants are immediately separated from their mothers, and many are sold as veal or banished to a dark, painful existence as a dairy cow.

Still another myth is that grass-fed cows are less likely to be contaminated by a food-borne illness like *E. coli*. Over a half-dozen recent studies have demonstrated that grass-fed cows are colonized with *E. coli* at rates nearly identical to grain-fed cows, and one study even suggested that grass-fed cows are more susceptible to *E. coli*.

Furthermore, just because there's a fancy "grass-fed" label on your beef doesn't mean it wasn't exposed to the same battery of synthetic chemicals as grain-fed cows. Shortly before they are slaughtered, all cows—grass and grain fed alike—are typically fattened up with corn and injected with artificial hormones.

Finally, even though grass-fed cows do enjoy a marginally higher standard of living than factory cows, grass fed will never be a viable alternative. According to the Humane Society, every year over 10 billion land-based animals are reared and killed solely for American consumption. That's 19,000 slaughtered animals every minute. That's 316 every second.

The only important difference between grass-fed and grain-fed meat is that one is hipper. If you slap a "grass fed" label on the package, you can charge ten bucks more for a product that lived under mostly the same circumstances and offers mostly the same nutrients as every other type of meat in the freezer.

Here's another way to look at it. We all know the nicotine in tobacco promotes lung cancer and other diseases. If a tobacco company came out with a line of "healthy, happy, organic" cigarettes, would you be fooled?

10

Craving Meat Isn't Natural

Here is another objection to a plant-based diet that comes up often: "If people shouldn't eat meat, why do we crave it?"

The fact is, there are times when craving something does mean you need it. When you're tired, you crave sleep, and you need it. When you're thirsty, you crave water, and you need it. Cravings are often signals to which we should listen. But is this true of *all* cravings?

Common sense tells us right off that not all cravings should be honored. An alcoholic craves alcohol. This is a self-destructive craving. A gambler craves gambling. A cocaine addict craves cocaine. Also self-destructive. These drives have been created by artificial, rather than natural, stimulation. Cocaine, for example, artificially causes the dopamine system (the reward center in the brain) to become hyperactive. Cocaine causes an artificial high that is more intense than humans were designed to experience, which is very dangerous, because once you experience it, you crave it again. This craving is the root of addiction.

All cravings were not created equal. Some, like cravings for water, food, sleep, and sex, are natural and normal and generally don't cause trouble. But cravings for unhealthy things can cause trouble.

What about cravings for meat? Are such cravings natural, or are they artificial? And if they are natural, does this mean that we should honor them?

Cravings for meat are, for the most part, artificial. To some degree this is because often people don't even crave meat when they think they do. For example, they may say they crave barbecued ribs, but those ribs have been ingeniously prepared with extra fat (oil, butter), salt, spices, and sugary sauce. When they say they crave chicken, they don't crave a piece of a bird. They crave something that has been fried in oil, and spiced up with salt or maybe a sugary sauce. In other words, most people's meat cravings aren't really for meat, but for a whole package of food that has been doctored up to become an artificial, high-sugar, high-fat, high-salt product. No wonder they crave it! Most meat is about as artificial as a donut or candy bar!

Is there any part of this meat craving that is real? I believe the answer is "no." Here's what my friend, eminent evolutionary psychologist Doug Lisle, says:

> Our ancient ancestors lived in a world where food was difficult to find. As a result, at some point in the distant past they evolved from a diet of plant foods to a diet that could accommodate some animal foods. Humans weren't designed to eat animal foods, but because of the threat of starvation, we adapted the capacity to use them. Think of cars that were designed to run on gasoline, but could also use alcohol. It wasn't a perfect fit, but it could work.

> When our ancestors started using animal foods, it caused problems because it wasn't the best fuel. It was *dirty* fuel. It clogged arteries, and it fed cancer. But at the time, this was better than starvation.

> Likewise, if you are dangerously dehydrated, you are not going to be very fussy about the cleanliness of any water you find. Even if it contains dangerous microbes, you will drink it. If you don't, you die.

> Similarly, it was a better move for our ancestors to include a dirty fuel, meat, into their diets than to starve. Better to live to sixty and die of a heart attack by eating some meat than to forgo all animal foods and have perfectly clean arteries but to die of starvation at forty.

> So our ancestors developed a modest craving for meat, not because they needed it, but because they needed to be forced to eat it if they were seriously hungry.

Fortunately, we don't face starvation today. So, if we're smart, we don't have to honor any cravings that encourage us to eat the dirty fuel.

In order to live long, live healthy, and prosper, we need to keep our diets clean and eat green.

Fact: Once you give up meat, you will stop craving it. People who've gone on the Engine 2 diet tell me that they couldn't believe that they would ever *not* want to have a burger. Today, just the thought of one makes them feel sick!

11

The Problem with Paleo

You've probably heard of the Paleo diet, in which people are encouraged to eat like a he-man or a she-woman cave dweller from Paleolithic times.

Here's what Jeff Novick has to say about this diet: If you are trying to eat as though you were a meat-eating cave person, then you're not following the best approach for optimal health through diet. Who's Jeff Novick? He's not just a good friend of mine, he's one of the country's leading dieticians and nutritionists.

So what's wrong with all the Paleo diets being promoted today? For one thing, our early ancestors didn't eat just meat. Up to 80 percent of their diet was actually plants. And it was these plants and the ability to cook starches and root vegetables that caused the great explosion in human growth and brain size.

The reality is the people in the Paleolithic Era ate more than 75 grams of fiber per day, or double that of the average plant eater today.

Next, it's estimated that the animal that would most resemble those consumed by Paleo types would be the antelope, whose flesh contains about 5 percent fat, hardly any of it saturated fat, and no added hormones or antibiotics—an animal far different from those that Paleo-pretenders eat today. (And don't forget that to eat a true Paleo diet, you'd also have to give up salt and sugar—which no Paleo dieter advocates.)

Interestingly, when researchers studied the hunter-gatherer tribes surviving today, they discovered that these people don't rely on meat at all—they eat whatever is available, and most of that is plants.

There are two populations today that still eat large amounts of meat. First, the Maasai tribe of East Africa, who basically live on blood, milk, and meat. Although many people think these people are free of heart disease, it's not so. In a study published in the *American Journal of Epidemiology*, Harvard's George Mann conducted fifty autopsies on the Maasai in the 1970s and found their bodies were loaded with heart disease—but unlike the arteries of Americans who eat a great deal of meat, the Maasai arteries were also dilated, allowing for more blood flow, due to their high degree of physical activity.

Second, the Inuit people in the northern parts of the Western Hemisphere eat a great deal of fish, blubber, and meat. Again, autopsy studies (done as far back as the 1920s) have confirmed the Inuit suffer from arterial plaque. In later research, American scientist Ancel Keyes also found the Inuits' arteries were severely clogged, their cholesterol levels high, and their bones weak because their high-protein diet had leached calcium from their bones. This demineralization was so severe that it was common for Inuits as young as forty to break a leg or hip bone while just walking. According to pathologist Arthur Aufderheide, "the spines of many [Inuit] women who died 8,000 years ago, nearly all before age forty, look like the hunched backs of eighty-five-year-old American women today."

If that doesn't turn you away from eating like Fred Flintstone, according to a major study designed to analyze the health and eating habits of more than 110,000 adults for two decades (published in the *Archives of Internal Medicine* in March 2012), eating *any* kind of red meat appears to "significantly increase the risk of premature death." Adding just one 3-ounce serving of unprocessed red meat to the daily diet was associated with a 13 percent greater chance of dying during the course of the study—and adding an extra daily serving of processed red meat, such as a hot dog or bacon, was linked to a 20 percent higher risk of death.

To defend their lifestyle, the Paleo people will often throw in the side argument that whole grains weren't part of the human diet in 100,000 BC. Well, neither were many other wonderful and healthful plants, such as broccoli, artichokes, lettuce, grapefruit, and most of the other produce we love today. And since countless studies have shown that increased consumption of whole grains is related to increased longevity and decreased obesity and heart disease, it's hard to argue against eating grains.

Don't rely on a speculative hypothesis to create your healthy diet. Rely on plants, and you'll be as strong as a caveman, and live three times as long.

Survey Says

At the end of 2011, *U.S. News & World Report* released its second annual ranking of the top twenty-five most popular weight-loss diet programs. The DASH (Dietary Approaches to Stop Hypertension) Diet, endorsed by the federal government, came out on top in several categories, including the lists of Best Diets Overall, Best Diets for Healthy Eating, and Best Diabetes Diets. At the drop-dead bottom of the list? The Paleo diet. The report notes that "Regardless of what a dieter's goal is—weight loss, heart health, or finding a diet that's easy to follow—most experts concluded he or she is better off looking elsewhere."

12

Eating Plants Is Easy

After traveling around the country for the last few years talking about the Engine 2 diet, I have heard just about every argument possible against a plant-based diet, and every excuse for not eating one. Excuses are like belly buttons—everyone has one.

A belly button that often comes up, usually at the very end of a talk, after all the others have been addressed, is this one: "But Rip, it's just too *hard* to eat a plant-based diet."

Come on, now! What's hard is *not* being healthy. What's hard is feeling run down 50 percent of your waking hours. What's hard is not being able to empty your bowels of little pebbles of bulkless, putrefying stools. Eating healthfully from a cornucopia of foods that come in all the colors of the rainbow and are filled with water, fiber, bulk, vitamins, minerals, plant chemicals, carotenoids, and antioxidants that promote exceptional health, energy, and vitality while keeping your dumps as regular as a Swiss commuter train is easy and fun.

Yes: It's super easy to eat a plant-strong diet, unless you're a troglodyte living thousands of miles away from all stores and without Internet access. For most people, eating plants is as easy as shopping at any market in America—not just health food stores, but also places known for their meat and dairy offerings.

Here are some easy tips for making the Engine 2 plant-savvy lifestyle work at any grocery store in America:

- **Make a shopping list with five columns:** whole grains, vegetables, fruits, legumes, and salt-free spices. If the item you're considering does not fit into one of those categories, there's a good chance you don't need it.

- **When you enter the store, turn right so you can start your shopping trip out in the produce section.** From there, go only to the sections of the store that you absolutely need to visit.
- **Avoid specialty products.** Even if you live in a larger city with a lot of shopping options, it is still important to keep things simple. Get the bulk of your nutrition from basic ingredients and whole, plant-strong foods.
- **Buy dry beans and grains in bulk when you can.** They will last a long time, and you won't have to worry about them spoiling, or about having to go out to buy new ingredients all the time.
- **If you'd prefer not to spend a lot of time cooking,** stock up on low-sodium (or no-salt-added) canned beans, quick-cooking brown rice (available most everywhere), and other quick cooking grains (quinoa can be cooked in about 10 minutes!). Keep a good supply of frozen vegetables and fruit around. This will make your life a lot easier when you find yourself without any fresh produce.
- **Buy just enough.** Too often you can get carried away by a sudden enthusiasm—due to clever packaging or a craving—for something you don't really enjoy all that much. Skip it.
- **Speaking of buying, buy what you like!** While eating a wide variety of fruits and vegetables can be fun, if you or your family just hate Brussels sprouts, then don't purchase them. If you love collard greens but hate kale, just buy more collard greens. As long as you are eating from those five simple food groups, you are going to rock it.
- **If you have kids, include them in the shopping process.** Let them help write the grocery list, pick out a few recipes they want to make, and choose a new fruit or vegetable for the family to try. My five-year-old son, Kole (named after the first half of my wife's last name, Kolasinski), and three-year-old daughter, Sophie, have become integral players when it comes to shopping for groceries, putting them away, and cooking our meals. It's a family affair!

Brick-and-mortar stores aren't the only place to get plant foods. Now that we live in the Information Age, take advantage of the Internet, where you can find all kinds of plant-based offerings available for overnight delivery, from simple and inexpensive basic foods to gourmet precooked meals.

For example, you can order tons of quality plant-powered products from Amazon.com. Check it out for nonperishable items such as dry beans, whole grains, and low-sodium beans. Another great website for ordering plant-strong products is vitacost.com. Check in periodically for sales, when you can stock up on some of your favorite sauces, canned goods, beans, grains, and hundreds of other products.

Of course, we all eat out sometimes, but that doesn't have to pose a problem. Many restaurant meals can be made plant-healthier with a few simple requests. Likewise, pizza restaurants that offer whole-grain doughs and plant-friendly sauces will also often accommodate a request for a cheeseless, meatless, veggie-heavy pizza with red sauce.

You're not going to get your best plant-strong food at a fast-food shack, though, because these places usually use white flour and processed ingredients. But if you have no other options, then eat as healthfully as you can. For example, at Chipotle Mexican Grill, you can do quite well by ordering the vegetarian burrito bowl and layering the bottom with three corn tortillas topped with brown rice, vegetarian black beans, bell peppers and onions, salsa, grilled corn, romaine lettuce, and guacamole.

Not long ago, I was in the Raleigh Durham International Airport and saw a sign for a burger joint, and I immediately thought, "Let me see if there's anything here that can accommodate a plant-strong guy like me." I looked at the menu and lo and behold, I found a vegetarian sandwich. And not just any sandwich. To a toasted bun without butter I was able to add as many items as I wanted from a list of great-looking vegetables. I went to town! Grilled onions, grilled mushrooms, jalapeño peppers, green bell peppers, lettuce, pickles, tomatoes, fresh onions, all topped off with barbecue sauce. It was terrific. And it cost a jaw-dropping $2.89! (Just be careful not to make these places your daily lunch spot, because even though they're great for fast food, their offerings are still cooked with oil and are high in calories.)

As you can see, the reality is that eating plant-strong in the twenty-first century in America is a piece of kale (not cake!). That's also why this way of eating is called the Engine 2 diet...it's just "2" damn easy, as opposed to "2" damn hard!

More Eating-Out Tips

I've traveled all over the country and have enjoyed plant-strong meals in all kinds of restaurants! When you're on the road, check online at http://happycow.net to find good places as you go. You can also download apps to your phone that will help you locate veg-friendly eateries.

Here are some ideas of what to order in different types of restaurants:

- **Asian restaurants:** Ask for brown rice, steamed vegetables, steamed edamame, or tofu, hold the extra sauces, and use low-sodium soy sauce sparingly. Another good option: brown rice vegetable sushi.
- **Italian:** Go for whole-grain pasta, tomato sauce (with no cheese added), and ask them to throw in as many grilled/steamed vegetables as they can find!
- **Steak house/American:** Believe it or not, you can get a great meal at a steak house. You can almost always find options like potatoes, sweet potatoes, and lots of steamed vegetables, or you can ask your waiter for a salad with every fresh vegetable they have on hand (and even fruit), with a side of balsamic vinegar (or sneak in your own plant-strong dressing).
- **Breakfast spots:** Request oatmeal made with non-dairy milk or water, fruit, and some nuts. You can also ask if they have whole-grain bread, a little nut butter, and fruit.
- **Coffee shops:** Hot herbal tea is always a great option. Most coffee shops carry non-dairy milk now as well instead of using dairy creamer. If you're having a snack, go for oatmeal. You can also get a little dried

(continued)

fruit and nuts at many places. I'm a frequent flyer for the Starbucks oatmeal in almost all airports.

- **Gas stations:** If you're on the road, you can find fruit at most convenience stores, and sometimes whole-grain pretzels or unsalted nuts as well.

- **Grocery stores:** Don't forget local grocery stores, where you can find items like oil-free hummus, whole-grain crackers or bread, cut-up and washed vegetables and fruit, cans of low-sodium beans (just be sure to pick up a cheap can opener). You can even buy potatoes and frozen vegetables to microwave later in your hotel room. Or you can make a great trail mix with whole-grain cereal, raisins, and a few nuts. Many grocery stores also have salad bars where you can make a great plant-strong meal.

- **At any restaurant:** Remember to watch out for processed foods and added oil. Ask if your meal can be cooked with vegetable broth, or steamed. Pei Wei, a chain of restaurants serving Asian-style dishes, is a good example of a place you can get a great plant-strong meal. You can order a veg dish with brown rice and ask them to cook it in vegetable broth in a style they call "stock velveted."

13

Eating Plants Is Thrifty

One of the biggest misconceptions about a plant-based diet is that healthy food equals expensive food. There are even some studies claiming to support this bunk. Their conclusions are based on a ridiculous "calorie per dollar" comparison.

The reasoning goes: There are more calories in a candy bar than in a banana, so candy bars are "cheaper"—even though bananas far outrank them in nutritional value. Well, if your only goal in eating is to throw as many calories as possible down the hatch every day, the calorie-per-dollar comparison would be perfect and you could live off of candy bars, hamburgers, and sugary sodas. You would also save money, because you would probably die before you hit forty.

Let's get real. Plant-based eating isn't more expensive than eating unhealthily; it's cheaper. And that's not even considering what you save in medical bills.

Seventy-two percent of Americans are overweight, and several estimates put the health-care costs related to this obesity at about $118 billion per year. Think about that the next time you buy so-called cheap meat. A report by the Worldwatch Institute found that obese people visit the doctor 40 percent more often than people of normal weight. These people are also two-and-a-half times as likely to need drugs for cardiovascular disorders. Even worse, overweight people are unable to work as much, with obesity accounting for 7 percent of lost productivity due to sick days and disability leave.

If you still think you save money buying unhealthy foods, think again.

When it comes to your shopping cart, you'll find that avoiding meat and eating plants will save you money as well as save your health. The beauty of a plant-based diet is that it doesn't rely on specialty ingredients like powders, exotic foods, or supplements. The healthiest, cheapest foods are sitting on your grocery store shelves; you just have to know what you are looking for.

I want you to eat like a peasant (beans, rice, fruits, and vegetables) so you can live like a king. If you eat like a king (meat, cheese, cakes, and pies), you'll get fat and sick and die like one. So saddle up, and let's take a money-saving and health-rescuing trip through the supermarket!

Here is a list of some of the cheapest plants you can buy:

Beans: Whether you call them a poor man's food or a smart man's food, beans are one of the cheapest and most nutritious proteins out there. At roughly 50 cents a pound for dried beans, they are almost giving them away. If you buy them dried, you'll have to soak them overnight, but at that kind of price, who cares?

If you're not keen on making your own beans from scratch, buy them in cans. Whole Foods Market carries several brands of no-salt-added varieties, including their 365 brand beans that are typically less than $1.00 a can. Not bad for a can of convenience and health rolled into one.

Oats: They are chock-full of fiber and complex carbohydrates, and cost about 50 cents a pound. The less processed the better, so avoid the flavored ones that look like flour and go for straight-up, old-fashioned rolled oats; or even better, steel-cut oats. Make a large batch of steel-cut oats on Sunday and store in the refrigerator for several quick breakfasts during the week.

Bananas: The power snack of the gods. Loaded with potassium and fiber, fat and sodium free, they're also great tasting—and all packed into one convenient travel shell. Bananas kick butt in just about every way: on top of the Rip's Big Bowl breakfast cereals, frozen and made into "ice cream" (see page 254 for a chocolate-banana ice cream recipe), in muffins (try the Mighty Muffins from *The Engine 2 Diet* book, which call for six bananas!), as an oil replacement in baking, and as a healthful, post-workout pick-me-up. The crops are susceptible to natural disasters, but as long as there haven't been any major hurricanes recently, bananas are sold for roughly 25 to 50 cents a pound!

Potatoes: Don't let all those nasty French fries fool you; there are good reasons why potatoes are considered a great staple food. They are full of vitamins and potassium, and they fill you up like nobody's business for about $1.00 a pound. Sweet potatoes are also a great source of beta-carotene. Eat your spuds well-washed, but with the skin on to get an extra boost of vitamin C and fiber.

And don't buy into the lore that potatoes are fattening or somehow unhealthy. The problem with potatoes is the company they typically keep—butter, sour cream, bacon bits—and the forms in which they're often found: sliced up in sticks and fried in oil, sprinkled with salt, and dipped in ketchup laced with high-fructose corn syrup. (Unfortunately, fries—those fat-, sugar-, and salt-laden sticks—are Americans' top source of vegetables!)

As a matter of fact, the potato won the award for vegetable of the year in 2008 from the WHO because it is such a plant-strong all-star. See pages 154 and 177 for mashed potato recipes, page 252 for a sweet potato soup recipe, and page 203 for a sweet potato burger recipe!)

Brown rice: At less than $1.00 a pound, all rice is a steal. But the brown stuff is full of stomach-filling, body-energizing, complex carbohydrates. Like potatoes, rice is also extremely versatile and can be thrown into anything from soups and salads to an outstanding veggie stir-fry, or even a delicious soy milk rice pudding. For added convenience, pick up a box of brown rice in quick cook bags. Simply throw a bag in a pot of boiling water and pull out 10 minutes later. No measuring and no fuss, only affordable convenience. Or check out the frozen section of any store for a three-minute brown rice, such as Whole Food Market's 365 brand or the new Engine 2 Plant-Strong™ whole-grain medleys.

But please, forget processed foods, even if they're plant based. A packaged dinner of pasta with tomato sauce will run you around $2.80 a serving at the grocery store. A family of four would be looking at spending at least $11.00 to feed themselves. For that amount of cash, they could make six servings of their own pasta with fresh ingredients and still be able to afford a salad and fruit.

Yes, there is a time commitment involved in preparing your own food. But if you compare it to the amount of time that people who eat unhealthily spend at the doctor's office for problems like obesity, heart disease, and diabetes, it doesn't seem like a waste of your precious hours after all.

Frozen Goodness

If a vegetable or fruit is not in season, buy it frozen. The price of frozen produce stays relatively stable throughout the year, even during the winter months when the price on the fresh stuff spikes. Nutritionally, frozen is similar, and sometimes even better than fresh produce. This is because it is picked at its optimal ripeness and then flash-frozen to seal in the nutrients. Some of the best frozen veggies are kale, peas, spinach, broccoli, green soybeans, and corn.

You won't find all of your favorite produce frozen, but according to the U.S. government's Federal Register, half of Americans' twenty favorite vegetables are also available in the freezer aisle. Avoid canned veggies when possible; the canning process sucks most of the good stuff out of them.

Here's a little trick with frozen vegetables. Thaw before you use them and then just warm them up in your dish as opposed to overcooking them. They've already been cooked, and cooking them twice makes them limp and diminishes their taste.

When it comes to fresh produce, it's best to buy it in season. A peach that was grown a few states away is going to be cheaper than one flown in from Chile. Also, the abundance of peaches on the market during the summer will keep prices lower until the end of the growing season. There is an added bonus if the produce is local and seasonal: It will have been picked at its ripest phase, giving it time to develop all the nutrients that don't exist in produce that has been picked early in order to ship it over long distances without rotting.

14

The World Is a Plant-Based Cornucopia

Here's one I hear all the time: "You don't eat meat? Then you must eat lots of tofu." Case in point: The first article ever written about us Engine 2 firefighters ditching flesh and flipping to plants was titled: "Tofu Outmuscles Red Meat at Firehouse." Nothing like perpetuating the myth about tofu. I mean, yes, we had some tofu here and there, but it wasn't like it was an everyday staple.

Meat eaters, omnivores, carnivores, and cannibals believe this myth because they developed their stereotypes about vegetarianism back when the "tofurkey" was still a novelty food...about thirty years ago.

I do eat tofu, but personally I'd rather chew on a shoe than eat it plain on a plate. The exciting thing about tofu is that it truly is a blank canvas that allows you to infuse it with or mold it into an infinite assortment of tastes, textures, and shapes. Whether it comes in a 16-ounce box in the dairy section in soft, medium, firm, or extra-firm, or in an aseptic, shelf-stable box, the array of possibilities that can be made from tofu is limitless: stir-fries, burgers, soups, desserts, dips, smoothies, stews, scrambles, and casseroles.

However, if tofu isn't your thang, there are several other dynamic, plant-meaty substitutes that might catch your eye and your palate, and save your heart.

First up, there's tempeh. If tofu is the ambassador of vegetarian proteins, tempeh is the James Bond: They do similar jobs, but tempeh just does everything with more style and effectiveness. Everything about it, from its nutritional content to its texture and its savory, nutty flavor, is bigger and bolder than its soy-based cousin. Tempeh also happens to be the only major traditional soy food that didn't originate in China or Japan. Instead, it comes from Indonesia, where it isn't just used for soups and stews, but is a staple protein.

Tempeh is made by inoculating cooked soybeans with a mold called *Rhizopus oligosporus* in a process similar to making yogurt. The soybean-mold mixture is then packed into cakes and left to cure into bricks of delicious, protein-packed goodness.

Tempeh contains about 37 percent protein, on average, which is about the same proportion as hamburger and chicken. It's also a great source of fiber, is easy to digest because it is partially fermented, and contains a measly 157 calories per 100 grams.

Oh, and did I mention that it's delicious? Whereas tofu needs to soak up other flavors in order to actually taste like something, the natural savoriness of tempeh means it adds flavor to dishes instead of just being a filler. It's perfect for stir-fries, barbecues, stews, and curries. Its firm texture also keeps it from crumbling into soy mash, as is often the case with plain tofu. (See the recipe for unbelievable barbecued tempeh sandwiches on page 168.)

If tempeh still doesn't have quite the bite you're looking for, try seitan. This Chinese invention is comparable to tempeh in nutrition but even more reminiscent of meat—so much so that some vegetarians refuse to eat it. It's made by kneading and washing wheat flour dough until all the starch has been rinsed off and you are left with a ball of pure protein, which is then simmered in flavored broth in order to set it and impart flavor.

At 81 percent protein and only 1 percent unsaturated fat per serving size, it's hard to beat this thousand-year-old "Buddha Food" for taste and nutrition. (See the recipes for an unbelievable seitan loaf on page 172, kabob on page 180, or Italian balls you can make at home on page 152.)

Most meat eaters operate under the delusion that if protein doesn't come from meat, it should at least act like it does. Quinoa doesn't care what anyone thinks: It's a seed (related to the beet and chard families) that looks and tastes like a grain but packs as much protein as meat.

Its goodness doesn't stop there, either: Quinoa contains nutrients including lysine, manganese, magnesium, copper, and phosphorus. No wonder the Incan Indians, who first grew it in the Andes around 5,000 years ago, called it the "Mother of All Grains." More recently, the United Nations designated it a "super crop." I just call it dinner.

The beauty of quinoa is its versatility; almost anywhere a grain will go, it will go better, so have fun with it. It can replace rice in a stir-fry or couscous in a salad. You can grind it up and put it in bread or cake dough, or even mix it with fruit and nuts and eat it instead of oatmeal in the morning. (See page 139 for The Machu Picchu breakfast and page 235 for the Red Quinoa Salad with Black Beans and Corn.)

A less versatile but still rib-sticking good protein source is a legume: the humble lentil. Humans have been eating these babies since prehistoric times (break that one out the next time someone hits you with the "our ancestors were meat eaters" argument), and lentils were long considered a poor man's food because they are cheap and nutritious. In my eyes, that also makes them a smart man's food.

Don't be fooled by the prejudices, though: Lentils are also one of the most flavorful of the legumes, and they are packed with more than 25 percent protein, folic acid, vitamins B and C, and both soluble and insoluble fiber. If that isn't enough, according to recent studies they are also super-troopers at helping to lower cholesterol. Eat them in soups, stews, and salads, especially during the winter, when you can really appreciate their hearty goodness. (See pages 176 and 190 for lip-smacking good lentil recipes.)

Next, don't let our fungi friends, mushrooms, fly under the radar! Low in fat, sodium, and calories, they are also packed with protein, fiber, antioxidants, minerals, and vitamins, and—when sunshine grown—one of the only food sources of vitamin D; 'shrooms have a terrific meat-like texture and are one versatile food. Have fun with portobellos slathered with barbecue sauce as burgers on the grill or sliced up and served with all the fixings as fajitas. Try sliding creminis or white buttons on a skewer with onions, bell peppers, and pineapples and build a killer shish kabob. Sprinkle them in salads for substance, toss them in stir-fries for flavor, mix them in with marinara sauces for texture, and strategically place them atop pizza for pizzazz! Or why not take a walk on the wild side and experiment with oysters, chanterelles, giant puff balls, morels, and porcinis? Mushrooms are a cornucopia of delectability!

Hey, and don't forget about nuts! They've got protein, fiber, and plenty of vitamins. One caveat, though: Because of the high fat and calorie content of nuts, limit your daily intake to 1 to 2 ounces (1 ounce is a small handful). The problem with nuts is that most people eat four to eight large handfuls in a sitting, and each handful contains approximately 200 to 300 calories! Before you know it, you've just tossed back up to 1,400 calories without making a dent in your tummy.

Personally, I use nuts as condiments to enhance my main meals rather than eating them as a snack food. I toss a small handful of walnuts on my cereal, pour a nut sauce on top of leafy greens (see page 216), sprinkle a mock nut-cheese on top of a pizza or casserole, add some nut spread to a sandwich (see page 171), use cashews in a pizza sauce (see the Arrabbiata Creamy Cashew Sauce on page 227), toss toasted walnuts on top of a salad, and even smear a little nut butter on my toast. As long as you avoid the sodium, sugar, and hydrogenated oils present in many nut butters, and aren't digging in with a spoon and bringing it straight to your mouth, I approve. Hey, we've all been there!

By the way, the foods mentioned above are just a few of the plant-based goodies in the repertoire. There are about, oh, 1,000 more we could talk about. Mother Nature's plant-based kitchen is about as large as, well, the Earth itself.

15

The Mediterranean Myth

Does this list sound healthy? Racks of lamb. Platters of fish. Bottles of red wine. Salads of feta cheese. Vats of yogurt. Ladles of olive oil.

Most Americans would say "yes" to these foods, which form the heart and soul of the so-called Mediterranean diet. And once you say Mediterranean diet, people think: "Wow, I can eat all these foods, do the Mediterranean thing, and live forever!"

The fact is, there is no real Mediterranean diet! Where did the myth originate? And why? And what's wrong with it?

In order to get the answers to these important questions, I asked Jeff Novick if he could lend me a lentil or two to help me get to the bottom of this riddle. We had a long conversation, and here's what we came up with:

First and foremost, at the heart of the Mediterranean diet is a multi-billion-dollar-a-year branding business that runs the gamut from hummus to packaged trips to Italy. It is a brilliant campaign concocted by the food industry, based on a lot of misinformation that even some of its proponents now admit was based on faulty research.

For one thing, there is no real Mediterranean diet. More than twenty countries border the Mediterranean Sea, and they have completely different diets. Some use olive oil, some don't. Some eat fish, some don't. Some devour feta cheese, some don't. Some drink alcohol, some don't.

According to Rami Zurayk, an agriculture professor at the American University in Beirut, "There is no such thing called the Mediterranean diet; there are Mediterranean diets...They share some commonalities—there [are] a lot of fruits and vegetables, there is a lot of fresh produce in them, they are eaten in small dishes, there is less meat in them. These are common characteristics, but there are many different Mediterranean diets."

In addition, in a 2009 article on dietary fat published in the *Journal of Clinical Lipidology*, author Dr. W. Virgil Brown (the journal's editor-in-chief) debunks the way the Mediterranean diet and olive oil have been promoted in the United States. He writes, "I'm afraid that this has become a great hoax applied to the American diet and that we have not paid as much attention to the data as we should have in order to make a better decision about the content of fat in our diet."

Let's take a good look at one of the countries that is supposed to be a sterling example of the great Mediterranean diet: Spain. According to one of the most comprehensive recent studies of Spanish nutrition and health, more than 50 percent of the 2,000 adults studied were either overweight or obese; 33 percent had high blood pressure; 65 percent had high cholesterol levels; and about 30 percent had three or more cardiovascular risk factors that could be modified by changes to their lifestyle or diet.

In regard to that study, Dr. Ricardo Gómez-Huelgas from the Internal Medicine Department at Hospital Carlos Haya in Málaga said, "The prevalence of obesity, diabetes, high blood pressure and high cholesterol in Spain have all risen at an alarming rate over the last twenty years and this is likely to cause future increases in bad health and death due to cardiovascular disease."

The myth of the Mediterranean diet seems to have originally arisen after World War II, when most people were still suffering the consequences of the war. Sami Zubaida, a leading scholar on food and culture, explains that back then, most of the area diets were similar in that they were composed of what the Italians called *cucina povera*: the "food of the poor." In the 1940s and 1950s, people ate lentils instead of meat because they had no choice. "A lot of it has to do with poverty, not geography," he says.

Here's what another expert, Dr. Anthony S. Wierzbicki, a London-based consultant in metabolic medicine, had to say: "The myth that the Mediterranean diet and lifestyle is so healthy is based on forty-year-old data from rural areas, and so much has changed during those four decades."

Case in point: The information that has been translated into the

Mediterranean diet originally arose from a 1950s study that found low rates of heart disease among people living on the island of Crete. While these people did consume some olives, avocados, olive oil, and other monounsaturated fats, their diets were predominately composed of fresh fruits, vegetables, whole grains, and legumes, plus small amounts of fish.

Part of the reason for this was that the community, recovering from postwar poverty, was very economically depressed and couldn't afford butter, cheese, and meat. As soon as they could, and did, they got fat. In fact, the rates of obesity and heart disease on Crete have been rising steadily since the time of the original study, as the Cretan diet and fitness patterns have changed. Visit the island of Crete today, and you will find obesity centers and billboards advertising gastric-bypass surgery strategically placed in downtown areas.

Still another study, from France, was also flawed: In 1999, the well-known Lyons study supposedly proved that the Mediterranean diet was better than a so-called low-fat diet. But when you looked at the facts, the people on the Mediterranean diet were actually consuming less fat, and much less saturated fat and cholesterol, than those on the low-fat diet! The latter diet wasn't really low fat. It was called low fat only because it was modeled on the current, typical American diet, which is lower in fat than the previous, 1960s typical American diet, which was 40 percent fat!

Don't be fooled by the marketing and advertising that is being pushed down our throats by the food industry. If there were a real Mediterranean diet, it existed at a time of postwar recovery and was a diet of poverty, limited resources, and food restriction. Today, more than half the populations of Italy, Portugal, and Spain are overweight. In eastern Mediterranean countries like Lebanon, obesity is looming in a large way. And Greece, the country most people think about when they think Mediterranean, is now the sixteenth-fattest country in the world, with more than two-thirds of its citizens overweight, according to a recent article in *Forbes* magazine.

So, for your best health, put down the olive oil (see chapter 29) and skip the hype about the Mediterranean diet. Instead, follow the time-honored and proven principles of healthy living and eating in practice all over the world where people eat a whole-food, plant-strong diet.

The French Paradox

The so-called French paradox is the belief that although the French eat a lot of meat and cheese, and drink a lot of wine, they have a low incidence of heart disease.

Just as he was able to show that there is no cure-all Mediterranean diet, my friend Jeff Novick can prove that there is no French paradox.

For one thing, the way that the American and the French medical communities account for heart attack differs substantially. As a result, many deaths that Americans attribute to heart disease are not counted by the French. In fact, 20 percent of these deaths are referred to as being from "natural causes." (Natural causes often being the result of consuming nature's most prominent fats, as in butter, cream, and meat.)

Another factor to consider is time lag. The research that supposedly backs up the French paradox was gathered over many years, but it's only in the last two decades that the French have really pumped up their intake of saturated fats and cholesterol-laden foods. When a new study comes out that investigates the relationship between the newly fatty French diet and heart disease between, say, 2000 and 2010, you'll see far different results.

In fact, according to a recent *Forbes* magazine survey, France is ranked as the 128th-fattest country in the world and climbing, behind Kazakhstan and Moldova. How often do you hear about the Kazakhstan diet?

Interestingly, one place where the French do show up as being healthier has nothing to do with *what* they eat but *how* they eat. A 2007 study from the *Journal of Obesity* asked American and French subjects how they know when to stop eating. In France, the top three answers were (1) when they started to feel full, (2) when they wanted to leave room for dessert, and (3) when they no longer felt hungry. Americans said (1) when they'd eaten what others thought was a normal portion, (2) when they ran out of a beverage, and (3) when the television show they were watching ended.

So the only real place where the French truly beat the Americans in terms of diet is that they are still listening to their bodies. They pay attention to their internal cues about when to stop eating, while Americans follow external cues.

Still, this wisdom isn't quite enough to save them from their increasingly bad habits: According to Inserm (the French National Institute of Health and Medical Research), research shows that from 1997 to 2009, obesity in French men and women increased 50 percent.

The big bottom line: When they eat like Americans, French women *do* get fat. So do French men, and French children, and, probably, French poodles.

16

Real Men and Real Women Eat Plants

Believe it or not, when Ohio Congressman Dennis Kucinich wanted to run for president in 2004, one of the reasons the press said he wouldn't be a viable candidate was because he is a vegan. That made him less than a real man.

For far too long, there's been a myth that real men and women eat meat. Part of the problem is wimpiness by association. People think of plant eaters as akin to thinkers and dreamers, not doers and fighters. The meat eaters have Genghis Khan, the plant eaters have Confucius. Ernest Hemingway gobbled up entire African game reserves, while Charlotte Brontë nibbled on salad. Ted Nugent will hunt anything that moves, while Moby wouldn't even attack a stuffed moose head.

This train of thought goes all the way back to antiquity. In Colin Spencer's *The Heretic's Feast: A History of Vegetarianism*, we learn that antiquity's greatest warriors were given the best cuts of meat, while its kings, like the famous Odysseus, were judged by the size of their livestock herds and their prowess in the hunt. Even the simple act of eating flesh was considered heroic. The great wrestler Milo of Croton is said to have consumed an entire bull while reclining in front of the altar of Zeus.

Meanwhile, the great thinker Pythagoras was a plant eater: He came up with the vital mathematical theorem about right-angled triangles that continues to be used by eggheads (and non-eggheads) everywhere. (In case any meat eaters out there have forgotten: In a right-angled triangle, the square of the hypotenuse is equal to the sum of the square of the other two sides. Or, $A^2 + B^2 = C^2$.)

Most of the famous plant eaters throughout history have in fact been thinkers rather than conquerors: Leonardo da Vinci, Jean-Jacques Rousseau, and Mahatma Gandhi, to name three. However, in Eastern cultures, there were some well-known tough-as-nails plant eaters, too, notably the Shaolin monks in the Henan province of China, who are among history's most celebrated martial artists. Similarly, many in Japan's samurai fighting class were vegetarians.

Today the plant-eating world is changing. More modern role models include Bill Ford (Ford Motor Company's executive chairman), Russell Simmons (hip-hop impresario), Biz Stone (Twitter Inc. co-founder), Mort Zuckerman (media mogul), Steve Wynn (Mr. Las Vegas), John Mackey (Mr. Whole Foods), and many more.

What do all of these highly successful business visionaries who are true early adopters know about a plant-strong lifestyle that 95 percent of Americans don't? They know the power of whole plants to control their health destinies. They don't want to play Russian roulette by eating meat, dairy, and refined garbage.

Many of these men and women have cited Dr. T. Colin Campbell and his book *The China Study* as a factor in convincing them to switch diets. Among them is former Kansas City Chiefs tight end, and current Atlanta Falcon, Tony Gonzalez, who read it in 2007. (His teammates nicknamed him "China Study.") It took some experimentation and some help from Jon Hinds, a plant-eating strength coach for the Los Angeles Clippers basketball team, but Gonzalez eventually settled on a plant-strong but not plant-perfect diet. By the end of the 2007 season, Gonzalez had broken the record for both touchdown receptions by a tight end and career receptions by a tight end.

If you want to read about more real men and women who decided to take their athletic performance to the next level with PEPFs (performing-enhancing plant foods), check out the next chapter.

17

Plant-Strong: The Athlete's X-Factor

When it comes to performance, athletes can be demigods. But when it comes to food, athletes can be scaredy-cats. They're often afraid of changing their diets because they think that change might hurt their performance. So they get stuck in the old status quo: Meat is good. Plants are bad.

Phooey! The truth is plants are the dope. In fact, plants are nature's legal performance-enhancing drug. I made the leap from a meat-weak diet to a plant-strong one in 1987, when I decided to become a professional triathlete. Plants gave me an abundance of phytonutrients, vitamins, minerals, protein, and water to support my body in its recovery phase after training and racing. Plants gave me clean carbohydrates that rapidly replaced depleted glycogen stores in my muscles and liver and allowed me to train harder, adapt, and improve. Plants gave me high doses of alkaline and anti-inflammatory substances that protected me from the stresses of four- to eight-hour training days. Plants gave me a clear head to focus like a laser beam. Plants gave me arteries and vessels that were youthful and elastic, improving blood flow to working muscles for killer oxygen uptake and enhanced VO2 max. Plants gave me a strengthened immune system that kept me healthy and free from illness. And plants gave me a lean and muscular body that was ideal for slicing through the water, pedaling efficiently in a time trial, and running like the wind.

This is not just me talking. According to study after study, the optimal athletic diet is very close to being completely plant based. If meat is included, it is present as an optional source of fat and protein, even for athletes who need to bulk up (and we all know there are better places to get your fat and your protein).

To understand why even the most serious exercisers don't need meat, you have to understand what an active body actually does need. All athletes, from triathletes like me to mixed-martial-arts fighters, require the same five nutrients to ensure they have plenty of energy: carbohydrates, fats, proteins, vitamins, and minerals.

Take a gander at that list: meat ain't on it.

Carbs are the most important food that an athlete can eat because they are the body's main source of fuel. Unlike fats and proteins, they are easy to digest and even easier to use when you need energy. Your body breaks down their starches and stores them in your muscles as glycogen, which offers hours of power for any kind of physical activity.

During the first hour of exercise, carbs provide half of the energy your body consumes. The harder you push it, the more carbs you use. The Academy of Nutrition and Dietetics (AND) recommends that athletes base 70 percent of their diets on this type of plant fuel, focusing especially on the so-called complex carbs, such as whole grains, starchy vegetables, and cereals.

Fat is your backup source of energy. Along with glycogen, your body metabolizes fatty acids for fuel, especially after the first hour of exercise. If you don't have enough, your engine will start to sputter. This is where most people turn to meat without thinking about what they are really putting into their body.

But the Olympic Training Center in Colorado Springs, Colorado, states that endurance athletes on high-carb, low-fat diets can actually perform longer than those on high-fat, low-carb diets. They get their fat from healthful whole-food sources like avocados, olives, oats, nuts, and green leafy vegetables (yes, green leafy vegetables contain roughly 9 to 11 percent healthy fat!).

Protein is another nutrient that people often confuse with meat. While many athletes (I'm looking at you, weightlifters) credit it as the secret to their strength, the truth is that most Americans eat too much of the stuff, which can lead to dehydration as well as tricking your body into not using the more efficient fuels available to it. Besides, you can't store protein as protein. If you eat too much, it turns into fat. All those protein shakes and supplements that people use to bulk up are just making them pack on unnecessary pounds.

The amount of protein athletes need is actually quite small, perhaps 10 to 12 percent of their total calories, according to the Academy of Nutrition and Dietetics. No one recommends that any athletes, even strength-training ones, eat more than 2 grams of protein per day for every kilo (2.2 lbs) of body weight. And remember, you can get all you need from plants like leafy greens, whole grains, beans, lentils, nuts, and seeds. (The Nevada state government recommends that even boxers get their protein from vegetable sources rather than meat.)

With their energy needs covered, a lot of athletes forget about fruits and veggies. Bad idea, says the Australian government, citing a 2005 study of athletes that found that not getting enough of the vitamins and minerals in fruits and veggies can lead to fatigue, muscle damage, and impaired immune function.

Heavy exercise makes you lose potassium and iron. You can re-up potassium on the go by munching bananas and oranges. Iron, which helps transport the oxygen in the blood to your muscles, isn't lost as quickly, so don't worry about trying to gulp down a can of spinach during a marathon. But do make sure to eat your leafy greens before and after exercise to replenish it. You can also boost your iron absorption by combining iron sources with vitamin C, as we talked about in chapter 5.

Exercise also stresses your immune system, putting you at risk of infection and disease. The vitamins A, C, and E, as well as the mineral magnesium found in fruits and vegetables, help guard against day-to-day illnesses that will run you down or even keep you out of the game. I'm not just talking about colds, either. Exercise causes the body to produce free radicals, those nasty particles that cause cancer, cell damage, and oxidative stress on the muscles. The best way to fight them is through antioxidants, and the best way to get those is through whole plants.

Study after study after study shows that the best source of antioxidants such as vitamins A, C, and E and selenium is whole, plant-strong foods and not supplementation. In fact, these studies suggest supplements of these nutrients in many cases cause more harm than good. Remember, the body doesn't know what to do with an isolated dose of these vitamins, especially when they don't arrive in a package it recognizes, such as an orange, apple, kale leaf, broccoli stalk, or sweet potato.

The list of athletes who have ditched the meat and switched to a primarily plant-strong diet to run their engines is growing like a garden of kale! Salim Stoudamire of the Atlanta Hawks basketball team doesn't believe in eating anything "that had a mother" and claims a steady diet of only plants has caused his endurance to go through the roof. Mixed-martial-arts fighter Mac Danzig won the 2008 season of Spike TV's *The Ultimate Fighter* eating brown rice, beans, soy, nuts, and vegetables—a diet pretty similar to that of the Shaolin monks. In addition to Danzig, MMA fighters Jake Shields, Herschel Walker, and James Wilkes have found the force in plants. The Williams sisters, Serena and Venus, are serving aces and winning tournaments with a daily protocol of plants, while former Heisman Trophy winner running back Ricky Williams and the newest NFL running back sensation, the Houston Texans' Arian Foster, are dashing through football defenses with plants. And Lizzie Armistead, one of Great Britain's best female cyclists and winner of a silver medal at the London Olympic Games in the relentless 87-mile road cycling race, is generating mega wattage by hailing to the kale.

Other famous athletes who kept their motors running with only biofuels are Basketball Hall of Famer Robert Parrish, tennis greats Martina Navratilova and Billie Jean King, the original strong man Bill Pearl, track and field Olympian Carl Lewis, bodybuilder Billy Simmonds, champion boxer and reformed ear-muncher Mike Tyson, winningest golfer of all time Gary Player, and the co–world record holder for number of Ironman triathlons won, Dave Scott, who also goes by "The Man." And then there's my friend John Joseph, whose form of athleticism takes place as the lead singer of the punk rock group the Cro-Mags, which means he gives performance after performance leaping around like a hyperactive banshee onstage, and diving off it into the crowd, for hours at a time—at the age of fifty!

How about the plant-strong supermarathon runners? Rich Roll, Brendan Brazier, and Scott Jurek (dubbed North American Male Ultrarunner of the Year from 2003 to 2005 and in 2007, respectively, by *UltraRunning* magazine) are crazy about plants.

Not long ago I was talking to Brazier, who recently wrote *Thrive: The Vegan Nutrition Guide to Optimal Performance in Sports and Life*, about the connection between plants and improved athletic performance. Here's what he told me: "Eating plants instead of meat gives you the edge as an athlete. For one, think about digestibility—you're not expending as much energy on food digestion. Then there's nutrition: You're getting more when you eat plants. And, there's less inflammation in a plant diet than an animal protein one, so you improve muscle functionality."

And when I asked Jurek, seven-time winner of the Western States 100-mile running race and recent author of *Eat and Run*, how making the switch to plants affected his performance, he replied: "I noticed changes in my body's ability to bounce back after hard workouts. Following a plant-based diet got me eating more whole foods, and because of that, my muscles don't get as sore and tired."

Although many of Jurek's and Brazier's competitors eat meat, there is another very special group of distance runners who don't. The Tarahumara Indians of the Western Sierra Madre in Mexico have been called "the finest natural distance runners in the world," and the most highly conditioned people "since the days of the ancient Spartans." Running is the primary means of transportation in their rugged mountain surroundings, and also a form of diversion. The traditional game of long-distance "kickball" sees individuals cover around 200 mountainous miles in two to three days. And they do it all on a diet of corn, beans, squash, and berries.

Two years ago, Christopher McDougall wrote the best-selling book *Born to Run*, which examined the Tarahumara culture, their plant-strong diet, and why they are the best endurance runners on the planet. Everything about these running Indians sounds far-fetched and fantastical, but I was lucky enough to see their world with my own eyes. In 2005, I went on a mountain-biking trip to the bottom of Copper Canyon (larger and deeper than the Grand Canyon) to an old silver mining town called Batopilas. On the twenty-five-mile ride down harrowing dirt roads (which required more than 6,000 feet of climbing on the way back!) I witnessed the Tarahumara living in caves on the side of the mountains, running down to the river to wash clothes or get water, and eating their plant-strong diets. It was a simple and magical world where time seemed to stand still and fantasy became a reality.

I asked Chris if he could tell me what these superhuman runners ate to fuel themselves during races. His answer: "I remember that we once made this great, 35-mile run—most of it straight up an incline. These guys would stop for a moment, take a long drink, reach into their pocket, and take out these little burritos that were a hand-made tortilla with a schmear of squash or beans inside. Then they were ready to go. When you're doing this kind of exercise, you want maximum energy and minimum effort processing it. They don't have much margin for error."

*   *   *

Hey athletes! Think of your body like a car. If you put in premium fuel, it will run longer and better than on economy unleaded. Meat isn't premium fuel. Maybe it does the job short term, but it comes with a lot of other baggage that isn't doing you any favors. And don't forget to fill up your tank, either. Athletes on plant-based diets are generally advised to eat 3,000 to 6,000 calories a day, while supermen like Jurek actually consume 6,000 to 8,000.

You might have to consume more than meat eaters, but a full tank of premium beats a quarter-tank of economy any day.

18

Lose the Moderation Mentality

Often, when meat eaters see that they are beaten, they fall back on the tried-and-tested diet rationalization "Moderation in all things." In other words, they're saying a plant-extreme diet is too much for nice, moderate people like them.

This phrase has been a favorite for eons. The Greek historian Hesiod said it way back in the ninth century BC. Aristotle also wrote about it. A version of it (*meden agan*, or "nothing in excess") was written on the Oracle of Delphi. The English poet Geoffrey Chaucer wrote: "In every thyng, I woot, there lith mesure." (For those of you who struggle with Middle English, me included, that means, more or less, "measure in all things"—but maybe you already wooted that.)

Chaucer lived to his mid-fifties. The ancient Greeks passed away, on average, at around thirty. So take a moment to consider the sources on this one.

The problem is that there are *some* things that should be abstained from completely. Whoever tells you it's okay to have a moderate amount of cocaine, or a moderate amount of heroin? A moderate amount of time sitting next to radioactive waste probably isn't very good for you either. Nor is moderate exposure to lead paint.

In fact, that little phrase, "Moderation in all things," is doing more damage than anyone could possibly realize.

Perhaps the best examples of foods we already know aren't good in moderation are the ones included in the fats, oils, and sweets section in the now defunct USDA food pyramid. They first appeared in the agency's recommendations in 1979, a result of American society's conquering malnutrition and becoming a nation that suffered from overeating.

In response, the U.S. government quickly shifted its focus from teaching people how to get enough nutrients to how to avoid the excessive food consumption that was causing chronic illnesses such as heart disease and stroke to skyrocket.

Contrary to popular belief, the inclusion of fats, oils, and sweets in the "Hassle-Free Guide to a Better Diet" (1979) was less an endorsement of "All things in moderation," and more an admission that "if you can't beat 'em, join 'em." They remained in the "use sparingly" category until the most recent incarnation of the USDA's food guide, where they have been abolished entirely.

Now, meat actually does have nutritional value. But let's look at the other things it has which you don't need in your body, even sparingly.

First, there is saturated fat, and plenty of it—it's part of what makes red meat taste so good. Unfortunately, it also causes obesity, raises your bad cholesterol levels, and, over time, clogs your arteries and promotes cancer.

Next, there is animal cholesterol. All animal products and by-products including skim milk contain varying amounts of cholesterol. Our bodies need cholesterol, but our liver makes all we need naturally, so we don't need to add more through our food. Red meat contains around 70 mg of cholesterol per 3-ounce serving, and chicken also contains 70 mg per 3-ounce serving—yes, they have the exact same amount! And meat eaters think chicken is healthier than red meat. What about fish, or eggs? Salmon contains 50 mg per 3-ounce serving, and 1 egg yolk contains 210 mg, which is the equivalent of the cholesterol found in two Burger King Whoppers! So, if you are trying to bring down your cholesterol and become heart healthy, you're barking up the wrong tree with any type of flesh, muscle, or meat.

Third, there is animal protein. Whether it's chicken, fish, or red meat, all flesh proteins create a rash of problems including raising our cholesterol levels, contributing to systemic bodily inflammation, draining precious calcium reserves from our bones, fertilizing and igniting tumors and cancer cells, and pummeling our kidneys and liver.

Next, let's look at what lurks in all the different dairy iterations, including liquid meat (milk), congealed meat (cheese), runny meat (yogurt), mottled meat (cottage cheese), and frozen meat (ice cream). The assassin hiding within all dairy products is casein, the animal protein that makes up about 86 percent of the protein in most dairy products. T. Colin Campbell, author of *The China Study*, refers to this animal protein as the number one chemical carcinogen in the American diet.

Fifth: In red and processed meats, you can find something called heme iron. Iron, of course, is an important mineral your body needs, but the type contained in meat has been linked to elevated levels of iron, which oxidizes in the body and contributes to inflammation, arthritis, diabetes, gallstones, hypertension, cancer, and heart disease. Plant foods contain non-heme iron, which is magically regulated by the body to prevent elevated levels and helps to prevent all of the aforementioned diseases.

Sixth: All meat and dairy increase what is known as insulin-like growth factor (IGF-1) production in the body. This is a "pro" growth hormone and leads to increased inflammation and is another cancer and tumor promoter.

Once you understand the insidious and destructive nature of the different elements lurking inside all animal foods and animal by-products, it makes it much easier to eighty-six the stuff in exchange for life-enhancing plants.

Another argument for dropping the moderation mantra is that by continuously feeding your palate these addicting foods, you are *never* allowing yourself to lose your cravings for these foods. And I mean that. Everywhere I go, people tell me they could never give up their cheese, their steak, their ice cream, or whatever because they love them too much. Is this love or abuse?

When I think of a loving relationship, I think of a mutual give-and-take, something that loves you in return. The reality is that cheese, steak, and ice cream do not love you back. They punish you with the contraband that is inherent in each of them. I am hereby letting you know you are officially in an abusive relationship, and as such I give you permission to sever the relationship. When you get home tonight, I want you to let these foods know you are finished with them. And when you kick them out of the house, be sure to tell them to not let the door hit them in the butt. You. Can. Do. It!!!

All kidding aside, maybe your mind can justify moderation, but heart disease doesn't know moderation, cancer doesn't respect moderation, type 2 diabetes laughs at moderation, and obesity and metabolic syndrome ridicule moderation. All these diseases begin at a cellular and molecular level, and all can be prevented and reversed at a cellular level with plant-healing food! Instead of nourishing disease it's time to nourish your health.

Mike's Moderation

Here's a well-written e-mail I received from a man who achieved excellent results following the Engine 2 program and wanted others to know the reaction he got from friends and family when they found out he was ditching the "Everything in moderation" mantra.

My wife's and my results have inspired a few folks to give the E2 diet a try, and I've had to warn them that they are going to be surprised how many scientist friends they have that they didn't know about.

It's amazing, really. I never heard a word of concern when somebody saw me eat my fifth piece of pizza after polishing off a plate of wings and a few beers. However, one word that I'm holding off on the meat and lowering my fat intake, and they come out of the woodwork.

They all seem to have kept their non-science office jobs, but suddenly they're evolutionary biologists talking about the shape of my teeth proving our omnivorous lineage, dietitians concerned about the exact percentage of my calories coming from protein, and biochemists who suddenly are worried about the details of my blood chemistry.

My advice? Smile, thank them for the advice, and ignore them like they ignored you when you were eating crap that was killing you. Then give them first dibs

(continued)

on your clothes before you take them to Goodwill because they are too big for you.

If they get excited about how I'm harming myself now that I've engaged in that horror of horrors—eating fresh fruits and vegetables!—I just tell them what they want to hear: It is very possible that this is just a fad diet that I'll stop doing sometime down the road, but if so, right now it is the most successful fad diet I've ever been on. So far, I've only seen positive effects from eating plant-strong. As soon as I see one single detrimental effect to my health, I'll reconsider my choice. I'll even give them the pleasure of buying me a nice juicy steak.

—Mike

19

Plants Are Eco-Friendly

Here's a simple piece of advice: If you care about the environment, stop being a carnivore.

Why? The sustainability gap between meat eating and plant eating looms as large as the Grand Canyon. Livestock farming requires far more space, energy, and water than agriculture. Even worse, it destroys its own resources through deforestation, overuse of land, and toxic runoff.

Every animal in the United States that is not raised in a field, butchered, and eaten by the same farmers who raised it requires huge amounts of fossil fuels to feed, house, kill, and transport it. For example, chickens need about 4 calories of fossil fuel for every calorie they offer. Eggs need 30, beef 35. That Easter lamb needs about 57 calories of fuel—that's about 6 gallons of gas!

If you average all of the meats, it takes about 25 calories of fossil fuel to produce every calorie of animal protein in America. In comparison, a calorie of plant protein requires only 2.2 calories of fossil fuel. You don't need to be Einstein to do the math on this one. According to the Food and Agriculture Organization, livestock production accounts for 18 percent of global greenhouse gas emissions—which is more than all of the world's automobiles combined.

So don't just bike to work and recycle your papers. Eat some broccoli!

A 2006 study from the University of Chicago estimates that the average American diet produces a two-and-a-half-ton carbon footprint every year, the same weight as a full-grown rhinoceros (who, by the way, is a plant eater!). A plant-based diet brings you down to a cool half-ton footprint.

Climate change too airy-fairy for you? How about deforestation? Chopping down trees to make room for supersize ranches is par for the carnivore's course. Look at what's left of the Brazilian part of the Amazon rain forest. A 2009 report released by the environmental group Greenpeace called cattle ranching the "primary driver" of deforestation in Brazil, with 79.5 percent of all deforested land being used for cattle ranches. It's a real tragedy that trees, one of our planet's greatest oxygen producers as well as filterers of pollutants, are being slaughtered without a second thought.

Aside from causing untold loss of biodiversity, cattle ranching has been responsible for nine to twelve billion tons of CO_2 emissions in the last decade in the Amazon region alone.

You can't lose trees without losing soil. Erosion destroys the ability of land to regenerate itself and eventually turns it into a lifeless desert. Farming is one of the leading causes of erosion in the United States, with 90 percent of farmland losing soil at a rate thirteen times greater than what's considered sustainable. Ranches and crop farms are both to blame, but erosion from plant farming happens at a rate six times slower than erosion from meat farming. Don't forget that most of those plants are going straight back to the livestock farm to fatten the cows.

It just gets worse, folks. The way meat destroys land is peanuts compared to the way it exploits water. One kilogram (2.2 lb) of animal protein requires one hundred times more water to produce than one kilogram of grain protein.

Livestock farms also pollute the same water they consume with pathogens like *Salmonella*, *E. coli*, *Cryptosporidium*, and fecal coliform, which seep into water tables, lakes, streams, and oceans. According to the Natural Resources Defense Council, more than forty diseases can be transferred to humans through manure. Translation: You don't want to be anywhere near this stuff in large quantities.

People living near cattle, pig, and chicken farms have found this out the hard way. In California, cattle farms and other types of agriculture are one of the major sources of nitrate pollution in roughly 100,000 miles of polluted groundwater. Nitrates have been linked to many issues, from increased rates of spontaneous abortions and blue baby syndrome to gastrointestinal problems and even cancer.

And then there are pig lagoons—cesspools of hog waste that often overflow and/or burst their banks when it rains. When that happens, you can kiss the nearest bodies of water goodbye. The 1995 bursting of one such lagoon in North Carolina released twenty-five million gallons of pig manure into the New River, killing about ten million fish and closing 364,000 acres of wetlands to shellfishing. (You might want to do a Google search to find out how far away you are from a pig lagoon.)

Even when it isn't causing fecal Chernobyls, everyday runoff from hog and chicken farms in Maryland and North Carolina is believed to be linked to outbreaks of *Pfiesteria piscicida* in the areas surrounding the farms, killing millions of fish and causing skin irritation, short-term memory loss, and other cognitive problems among those humans unlucky enough to live near these farms.

The only creatures in the world that really groove on fecal and fertilizer runoff are algae. In the Chesapeake Bay, algal blooms due to farm runoff have caused the crab population there to drop by 70 percent. In the Gulf of Mexico, the blooms have created a dead zone (where not enough oxygen is present to support aquatic life) roughly the size of Connecticut.

What about seafood, then? According to a recent United Nations Environment Programme (UNEP) report, 72 percent of the world's marine fish stocks are being harvested faster than they can reproduce. On top of that, 25 percent of the total yearly catch is made up of bycatch, i.e., waste fish that usually die. In 2003, that amounted to roughly 27 tons of "waste." Halibut fishing is one of the worst culprits: 95 percent of the fish it pulls in are bycatch, including a fish market's worth of endangered or overfished species.

In 2006, a group of scientists from five different countries studied the viability of the world's marine fisheries. Their conclusion? If catch rates continued unabated, the populations of all currently fished species would collapse by the year 2048.

That's just thirty-five years from now.

Agriculture ain't perfect. In a 2003 report, leading environmental scientist David Pimentel of Cornell University wrote that neither meat nor plant-based diets were sustainable given current farming practices. But we can't stop eating altogether, so the best way to limit the environmental impact of farming is to cut out the farming that takes the heaviest toll. The average American consumes around 200 pounds of meat a year. When you consider that producing one pound of "factory-farmed" beef requires seven pounds of grain and 2,400 gallons of water, it's easy to see where to begin.

In my opinion, eating meat or fish after you've read about the impact it has on the planet is as appalling as driving around a gas-guzzling Humvee instead of doing what you can to lighten your carbon footprint. It's time to stop growing plants only to feed animals and start growing them to feed ourselves. Eat some Swiss chard today and save the world tomorrow!

20

Avoid Contamination.
Eat Plants.

Question: Where's a good place to find contaminants, besides in your garbage can and your local dump? Answer: In meat!

All those pesticides, heavy metals, antibiotics, and other toxicants floating around farms accumulate in the fat of animals and enter your body when you eat them. The list of contaminants that can be found in meat reads like something out of a meth lab: arsenic, lead, ammonia, copper, penicillin, nitrites, and the scariest: ivermectin, a neurotoxin that can actually kill your brain cells.

Those are just the beginning. There are so many contaminants in meat that no one is sure exactly how long the list has gotten. The FDA estimates that it contains between 500 and 600 different unnatural chemicals.

Unfortunately, the government only tests for sixty of them. Among the ones that they *don't* test for are most carcinogens, chemicals that cause birth defects, and some dioxins, a class of ultra-nasty toxicants that is linked to reproductive and developmental problems, immune system damage, and, of course, cancer. More than 90 percent of human exposure to dioxins is through meat.

The United States General Accounting Office puts the number of possible contaminants a little lower, at precisely 143. Of those, forty-two can cause cancer, twenty are linked to birth defects, and six, according to the *New York Times*, "are suspected of causing mutations." Even the USDA, which is supposed to be protecting consumers from these poisons, has admitted twice that it has failed in its job to monitor them.

In his book *Diet for a Poisoned Planet*, David Steinman estimates that 90 to 95 percent of all the toxic chemicals humans ingest come from meat, fish, dairy, and eggs. On top of that, meat contains fourteen times more pesticides than plants do, and dairy has five times more. Although plants can also contain contaminants, they aren't treated with, and exposed to, the same number as animals are, nor do they store the toxic substances in the same way.

Farm animals are bombarded with toxicants every day: They eat food containing pesticides, they take drugs to make them grow faster and keep them healthy, and they may even drink water that has been accidentally contaminated with fertilizers and heavy metals. All of this "shawowzie" is stored in their fat deposits, where it accumulates until meat eaters unknowingly consume it.

Some of the toxicants in animals that are turning up in meat aren't even legal and some haven't been used for thirty years. They are called Persistent Organic Pollutants (POPs), and range from pesticides like DDT to industrial coolants (DDT has been linked to cancer, miscarriages, and infertility while coolants are linked to diabetes). Even though most were banned in America in the 1970s and 1980s, their residues are still hanging around in the environment. A new class of toxic flame retardants is also ending up in our bodies; these have been shown to disrupt the functioning of healthy endocrine glands.

By the way, you fish fans: It's not just furry animals that contain these poisons—a 2004 study found the highest levels of coolants in farmed salmon.

One reason that toxic chemicals remain in the food chain is because factory farmers feed their animals what's known as "litter," a slurry of feces, dead animals, fur, feathers, and feed remnants that were themselves contaminated; this litter has been linked to all kinds of things from mad cow disease to food poisoning.

According to the USDA, contaminated animal flesh is the cause of 70 percent of food poisoning cases every year. One of the biggest culprits is natural but nasty: a little guy called *E. coli*—a normally helpful bacterium that lives in our intestines but can wreak major havoc if we ingest it. Despite causing tens of thousands of cases of food poisoning every year, it was actually legal to sell meat tainted with *E. coli* until 1994, when a massive outbreak via a chain of popular fast-food restaurants killed four kids.

E. coli gets onto animals when they are in contact with feces, and it remains there when they are slaughtered and their flesh turned into meat. It is often cooked off, except in the case of hamburgers; this is because they are a putrid mash of fat, gristle, and low-grade cuts of meat mixed up and formed into a patty. You might cook the *E. coli* dead on the outside, but the inside might still remain contaminated. According to the *New York Times*, many big slaughterhouses refuse to sell meat to grinders who test for *E. coli*.

Unfortunately, the response by the meat industry to these issues hasn't been to improve standards but to pump their animals full of still more toxic chemicals. In order to get rid of *E. coli*, some meat producers treat it with ammonia—the same stuff that's in your window cleaner. Meanwhile, many chickens are kept bacteria-free with food that contains arsenic, one of the most toxic natural substances known to man.

If an animal is turned into processed meat—hot dogs, bacon, luncheon meat, or basically anything on a club sandwich—its flesh is pumped full of nitrites as a way of preserving, flavoring, and coloring it. The problem is that nitrites can combine with the meat's amino acids during the curing process to form nitrosamines, aka carcinogens. A study by the World Cancer Research Fund and the American Institute for Cancer Research (AICR) found that a person's risk of getting colorectal cancer increases by 21 percent for every 50 grams of processed meat consumed daily. That's just one hot dog!

To add insult to injury, meat won't only make you sick, it will keep you from getting better. Many beef farmers give their cows antibiotics at what doctors call "sub-therapeutic" levels. In plain English, it's not to cure them of disease, it's to make them grow faster. It's been estimated that farmers use fifteen to seventeen million pounds of antibiotics every year just fattening their cows.

And what happens to germs when they see the same antibiotics over and over again? They become resistant to them—bad news if *you* need some antibiotics to actually fight an illness. Doubly bad news if you got that illness from meat, which is often contaminated with antibiotic-resistant strains of bacteria. There is even some evidence that antibiotic resistance can be transferred by eating meat. In 2010, the FDA issued a warning to meat producers saying that dosing cows was "a serious public health threat."

With 99 percent of the meat in America coming from factory farms, you can never be sure of its quality, or how the livestock it comes from were raised. The one thing you can always bet on is that it will be oozing toxic substances that have no business being in it, or in you.

21

Chocolate! You Bet!

Adopting a plant-based diet means giving up some foods you're fond of. When President Clinton started following my father's program to reverse heart disease, he had to ditch fried chicken and cheeseburgers, which for a stubborn Southern boy like him was almost like telling a bear to give up honey.

That doesn't mean you have to give up everything you love. Some of your favorite, most delicious, most satisfying, and seemingly sinful foods aren't necessarily bound for the compost heap along with the pork, turkey, milk, and ice cream. What foods, you ask? Well, how about 70 percent or more dark chocolate!

Some of your animal-eating friends may assume that chocolate bats for their team because it tastes so good, but the truth is that dark chocolate, in its purest and most natural form, is plant based.

Unfortunately, some of the junk that passes for chocolate today is so refined and stuffed with so many additives that it more closely resembles a frightening science experiment than an actual chocolate treat. Take a look at the ingredients label on a typical candy bar. You may not have noticed it, since it's cleverly concealed in tiny print behind that plastic flap. For something like chocolate, there are a heck of a lot of ingredients that don't sound very chocolatey, such as cornstarch, lactose, dextrin, titanium oxide, and lots of milk fat.

One of the cheapest and least pure forms of chocolate—the stuff you find in most candy bars—is packaged milk chocolate. Some of these products contain so little actual chocolate that they have to stuff them full of artificial flavoring and milk fat just to give them some taste. The result is an extremely fattening chunk of chemistry that offers almost no nutritional value.

Dark chocolate doesn't have as many ingredients. It is derived from the pods of the glorious *Theobroma cacao* tree—or cocoa tree for short, and generally contains chocolate liquor, cocoa butter, cocoa powder, and a sweetener.

Chocolate is an excellent source of antioxidants, which support all kinds of health. And new research has shown that naturally occurring cocoa phenols can discourage plaque buildup in your arteries. Studies have found that the health benefits of chocolate increase dramatically with its purity; in other words, the more chocolatey and plant-based the chocolate, the better it is for you!

So make sure you check the label closely when buying chocolate. Lots of brands try to pass themselves off as "dark" or, my personal favorite, "all natural." Make sure there's no added milk, and apply the general rule that if you have a hard time pronouncing the ingredients, or it takes a while to read through all of them, it's probably not real chocolate.

When Bill Clinton appeared on the David Letterman show in 2011, Letterman asked Bill why he looked so good, and Bill mentioned his plant-based diet. Letterman remarked he didn't want to give up meat and dairy and that he had a tendency to "fudge" too much. Bill responded that speaking of "fudge," even the most militant plant-based eating doctor, Dr. Esselstyn, would eat some chocolate every New Year's Eve. Letterman responded with "Wow! He goes crazy New Year's Eve!"

The truth is my father does eat some chocolate every New Year's Eve. But it isn't just a little bit and it usually isn't even dark chocolate. He has between twelve and fifteen Reese's peanut butter cups!

No one is saying that a lot of dark chocolate is healthy—it has too much fat and can contribute to weight gain in a hurry. Don't go out and eat a bunch of chocolates now. But what I am saying is that the plant-based world is filled with wonderful treats, whether it's ripe tropical fruits, creamy rich nuts, or, yes, even a little lip-smacking good chocolate now and then.

22

Plants Perk Up Your Pecker

Question: What disease will kill one out of every two men and women? Answer: Cardiovascular disease. Question: What is the first clinical sign of heart disease in men? Answer: Erectile dysfunction. That's right. The canary in the coal mine when it comes to male heart disease is an underperforming penis. What's the best way to avoid it? Is it by downing handfuls of red meat? No! Is it by downing handfuls of blue pills? No! The best way to perform in bed is by downing handfuls of leafy green vegetables and whole plants.

The idea that meat is good for sex is just another in a long line of medical myths. For example, the nineteenth-century dietary crusader Sylvester Graham (famous for the cracker named after him) thought that meat encouraged "sensuality." Even odder, English schoolteachers in the early twentieth century told their pupils to skip meat in order to reduce their urges to do what teenage boys do when they are alone. Fat chance of that!

Another school of thought was that impotence was caused primarily by psychological issues, and that eating meat made the male ego stronger and, therefore, more psychologically fit to get sexually aroused.

Wrong on all accounts. Doctors now believe that around 85 percent of impotence issues are caused by medical or physical problems. And for the thirty million American men who suffer from erectile dysfunction, meat is actually part of the problem. Why?

What makes an erection really great is good blood flow. When men become aroused, their bodies release a chemical called nitric oxide that has the same effect on their Johnson that nitrous oxide has on a car: It supercharges it. Blood flows to the penis and increases it to roughly twice its normal size, and, just like that, you're off to the races. But you won't be racing anywhere if your blood isn't racing down there.

Says Terry Mason, the chief medical officer of the Cook County Health and Hospitals system in Illinois, about a discussion at a 2010 joint meeting of cardiologists and urologists at the National Medical Association convention, "We found [a] strong relationship [between erectile dysfunction and a fatty diet]...due to damage to the endothelial cells. The endothelium is the thin layer of cells that line the interior surface of blood vessels. Now, the penis has more endothelial cells per unit volume than any other organ in the body. So anything that would affect endothelial cell function would be a problem in the penis."

That's where meat comes in. Obesity, heart disease, atherosclerosis, and high blood pressure caused by diets high in saturated fats, cholesterol, animal protein, and processed foods are the major causes of impotence in the United States. According to a recent article in the *New York Times*, more than 40 percent of impotent men suffer from hypertension. If your arteries are blocked from too much crap, the amount of blood flowing through your body is reduced, meaning there isn't enough to pick you up when you want to get down.

To help you understand why the artery to the penis tends to block up first and foremost, let's take a look at the diameter of two arteries. The coronary artery that flows to the heart is about 5 mm wide, or the size of a normal drinking straw. The artery to the penis is a mere 1 mm wide, or the size of a little coffee-stirring straw.

Which one do you think would clog up quicker? Makes you think, doesn't it, guys?

A study of 3,000 men by the National Institute on Aging found that men with higher blood pressure had double the risk of developing a useless tool between their legs than those with lower blood pressure.

These discoveries have also debunked the old impotence myth that men lose their sex drive as they age. In 2007, the *New England Journal of Medicine* published a report on the largest sex study of seniors ever conducted; it showed that healthy old timers often feel as frisky as anyone else. It's the sick ones who need a little pill. Doctors now believe that older men lose their mojo because they are more likely to have diseases that compromise their blood circulation, like heart disease, diabetes, and high blood pressure, all results of eating too much meat.

In other words, going flaccid is not a natural part of the aging process.

All this is good news for plant-strong eaters because if a food is heart healthy, it is also pants healthy. So if you want to keep raising the flag, snuggle up to libido-friendly fruits and veggies. Foods that come from animals just clog your arteries and keep blood from flowing to the place you need it most: your Eiffel Tower.

23

Veggies Give Verve
to Your Vulva

Not long ago I received this testimonial from a new adapter to the plant-strong life who happens to be sixty-nine years old. "Dear Rip: Sorry to make this R rated. But I have to tell you I have been on plant-based eating for about 11 months now. I am 100 pounds lighter. I am 69 years old and I have not had sex for years with my husband. The last month I just can't get enough of him. I am convinced the blood flow has reached new and exciting places, thanks to the Esselstyns' books and DVDs. It's like getting married all over again."

It's true for women as well as men! Plants improve your enjoyment of sex. To prove it, I have handed over the reins for this chapter to my sister, Jane Esselstyn. Jane has been teaching sex education to middle-school boys and girls for more than eighteen years using an open, humorous, and approachable style. She's also a mother of three, writes a blog called *Puberty from Head to Toe*, and is a plant-strong cooking genius. Take it away, Jane!

For women, the term "sexual health" could simply refer to a rocking, healthy sex life, but it also refers to her body and the systems associated with her gender: breasts, uterus, endometrium, body fat, and vascular system. Most people don't realize that applying a plant-strong diet to the complicated equation of women, sex, and health engenders exciting results.

As discussed in the previous chapter, a major benefit of eating a plant-based diet is blood flow. Blood flow is essential for a penis to achieve an erection. Similarly, blood flow helps women in different areas, in different ways.

Front and center in this blood-flow discussion is the clitoris. In GPS terms, this little bundle of eight thousand nerves, this doorbell of desire, resides just south of the pubic bone, just ahead of the vaginal and urethral openings, and is housed between the genital labia (lips).

The clitoris is only the beginning of the story. This external button is literally only about one-tenth the size of the equipment within. When a woman is aroused, the external clitoris, also known as the glans, engorges with blood. Not as much as a penis, but more than you'd imagine, for as the romantic mood and physical stimulus continue, the *internal* clitoris starts to engorge, as well.

This tissue, called the *corpus cavernosa*, is the same engorgeable tissue found within the penis shaft. Blood flow into the internal clitoris causes engorgement and deeper arousal. Blood flow here is not insignificant, because the full range of the internal clitoral tissues, the *corpus cavernosa*, is intriguing: This tissue lassos around the vaginal space. In other words, when engorged with blood from well-dilated vessels, the arm-like clitoral *corpus cavernosa* tissues reach around the vagina like a snug hug.

At the same time, the brain's arousing messages trigger the vaginal walls to lubricate. Where does this lascivious lube come from? Blood flow. Vessels carrying blood to the vaginal walls literally seep plasma through the vessel walls, creating friction-free vaginal lubrication. This critical blood flow can only be ensured by a plant-strong, meat-free diet.

Blood flow aside, I would think that some of this woman's sexual behavior may well stem from her weight loss and empowerment now that she feels better about who she is and how she appears to herself and others. Body image is a big deal when it comes to sexuality. If you feel good in your body, you feel comfortable being sexual with your partner.

If you do not feel comfortable with your sexual self, you can create barriers. Some people tend to judge themselves in a critical way during a sexual experience. This behavior, identified by sex researchers Masters and Johnson decades ago, is called "spectatoring." It's as if one is a critical audience of oneself. This behavior prevents the mind from "getting into it." The brain has to send signals from up above in order for things to get flowing down below, and without the blood flowing, tissues engorging, cuffing outside of and lubricating within the vagina, the encounter is not going to feel like a positive, healthy, sexual experience.

So eliminate spectatoring and delight in what your body can do. Eating plant-strong will make you feel great within your body, and you'll be bombarded with compliments on your fine new plant-strong figure. All of which allows blood to flow full steam ahead!

And they say broccoli isn't sexy!

24

It's Never Too Late to Start a Plant-Based Diet

I first met eighty-year-old Darrell Williams when he wrote me a letter after one of his friends heard me speak to a Boy Scout troop. I thought Darrell would enjoy my plant-strong message, so not long afterward he and I drove to Southwest Texas State University, where I spoke to a hundred college students. Along the way Darrell told me his story.

For most of his life, Darrell knew and cared little about nutrition, even though he taught physical education at the University of Texas. He ate the average American diet: pizzas, burgers, dairy, and processed foods. His weight ballooned from 163 in college to about 230 by the time he was age sixty. He never felt well, suffering from ulcerated colitis, elevated blood pressure, severe allergies, hemorrhoids, irritable bowel syndrome, kidney stones, and severe backaches.

Then, in his late sixties, Darrell saw a doctor who suggested he stop eating dairy. He did, and the allergies disappeared. Darrell became more interested in the relationship between diet and health, eventually reading many books on the subject. That's when he looked me up.

Today Darrell eats the Engine 2 way: fruits, vegetables, legumes, and whole grains. His weight is down to 170. His blood pressure is excellent. He no longer suffers from all his ailments. He feels great, but the best part, he says, is actually what he *doesn't* feel anymore: the aches, the pains, and the cramps. "All my life I felt like my body was getting in my way. Now, it feels invisible—it's never in my way."

Darrell is a true Renaissance man who not only has done a 180 with his diet, but also has taught himself how to play the piano and guitar, and he is an avid reader on all topics. Darrell's zest for living is the how and why behind the change he made in his diet and lifestyle. And it is also why he has become one of Jill's and my closest friends and a surrogate grandfather to our kids!

Darrell also proves that it's never too late to start a plant-based lifestyle! A rich diet of fruits, vegetables, and whole grains can even reverse the onset of chronic diseases like high blood pressure, diabetes, and heart disease.

That's important, because according to the American Heart Association, 82 percent of all fatal heart attacks occur in people older than age sixty-five. Consistent meat-munching and milk-guzzling leads to the accumulation of plaque in the arteries, as well as those dangerous little gel plaques leading to the heart and brain that cause heart attack and stroke.

Moreover, many seniors erroneously believe that their cancer risk isn't affected by age. But the truth is that nearly four out of five cancers are diagnosed after age fifty-five, and by sixty-five an individual's cancer risk is ten times greater than in his or her youth.

However, as the American Institute for Cancer Research (AICR) has noted, "You can't control your age, but you can control your cancer risk." In fact, the AICR recently launched an awareness campaign called "It's Never Too Late to Lower Your Risk." The campaign encourages seniors to exercise regularly and, most importantly, to adopt a plant-based diet.

The excess weight we tend to carry in our later years can actually increase our cancer risk. Fat cells—both the unsightly belly kind as well as the visceral fat that lies deep in the abdominal cavity and pads the spaces between our abdominal organs—cause an imbalance in our hormones that can lead to insulin resistance, low-level chronic inflammation, and excessive production of estrogen, which in turn promotes cell growth. The faster turnover rate of cells increases the chances that cancerous mutations can occur. As the AICR notes, "maintaining a healthy weight may be the single most important way to protect against cancer."

For seniors, the AICR advises that all meals be based on plant-based foods. A consistent diet of fruits, vegetables, and whole grains will "protect against a range of cancers, including mouth, pharynx, larynx, esophagus, stomach, lung, pancreas, and prostate." Apart from providing all the vitamins and minerals our body needs, a plant-based diet is an excellent source of glorious little chemicals called phytochemicals, which discourage cell mutations and, therefore, lower our cancer risk. Think of antioxidants and phytochemicals as little fire extinguishers that activate over free radicals and neutralize them from doing damage and instigating cancers. Or as Dr. William Li (president, medical director, and co-founder of the Angiogenesis Foundation) put it, fruits, vegetables, and whole plant foods are nature's anti-cancer foods, our "culinary medicine." Nature's own form of chemotherapy and radiation!

25

It's Never Too Early to Start a Plant-Based Diet

You've just read about the benefits of starting a plant-based diet in your later years. But why wait for all that meat and dairy to beat up the body before making the switch? Why not start as early as possible?

No doubt about it: Kids who are raised on a proper plant-based diet will be setting themselves up for a lifetime of sensational health. As the Physicians Committee for Responsible Medicine (PCRM) notes, "Children raised on fruits, vegetables, whole grains, and legumes grow up to be slimmer and healthier and even live longer than their meat-eating friends," while "children who acquire a taste for chicken nuggets, roast beef, and French fries today are the cancer patients, heart patients, and diabetes patients of tomorrow."

An interesting tidbit: Back in 1924 at Yale Medical School, the cadaver-dissecting partner of my grandfather, Dr. Caldwell Esselstyn Sr., happened to be none other than Benjamin Spock, who'd eventually write *The Common Sense Book of Baby and Child Care*, one of the seven top-selling books of all time. In the last edition of his world-famous book, produced while he was alive, Dr. Spock says: "We now know that there are harmful effects of a meaty diet...Children can get plenty of protein and iron from vegetables, beans, and other plant foods that avoid the fat and cholesterol that are in animal products." As for dairy foods, Dr. Spock writes, "I no longer recommend dairy products after the age of two years. Other calcium sources offer many advantages that dairy products do not have."

Parents don't knowingly put the health of their children in jeopardy, but the sad effects of an animal-centric diet are not immediately apparent. We know that prolonged consumption of saturated fats and cholesterol promotes heart disease, diabetes, and countless other chronic diseases. We know certain cancers are directly linked with animal-based diets. Yet far too many children are being raised on an unhealthy lifestyle that becomes increasingly difficult to kick, and will one day jeopardize their health.

In fact, nutrition expert Dr. Joel Fuhrman asserts, "When the data is reviewed with completeness and integrity, one has no choice but to recognize that the diets most people are feeding their children today must be seen as child abuse. They destine their child to a lifetime of compromised health and a premature death from cancer."

While nowadays I can't imagine anything more delicious than a bowl of sweet brown rice, perfectly sautéed vegetables, and a steamin' hot plate of seasoned black beans, kids who have grown up guzzling cherry coke and bacon burgers might have trouble adapting to a new diet. But all kids can change. For example, before 1985 my family ate just as much American steak and cheese as anyone. Then, when my father discovered the plant-based secret to long-lasting health, all of us Esselstyns switched our diets. It was easy and fun, and the family's plant-tastic voyage is now in its third generation as my children, as well as my nine nieces and nephews, are all happily eating plants.

After all, all the essential vitamins and nutrients that kids need to grow can be found in a plant-based diet. Instead of raising your child on animal products, which are high in the trifecta of saturated fats, cholesterol, and animal protein, try a mixture of whole grains, legumes, vegetables, and fruits that offer healthy fats, zero cholesterol, and friendly plant protein.

For growing children, steady sources of vitamin B12 and calcium are important. Many plant milks, from oat to almond, are fortified with a bountiful supply of both, and plenty of calcium can be found in lentils, beans, peas, sweet potatoes, collards, kale, mustard greens, Swiss chard, and other green vegetables. A steady source of iron is also crucial, and can be found in lima beans, red kidney beans, black beans, split peas, potatoes, broccoli, spinach, kale, rice, raisins, sesame seeds, and walnuts. Iron absorption is maximized when paired with the abundance of vitamin C found in fruit.

For younger children, PCRM recommends a slightly higher fat intake. But remember, not all fats are created equal! Most American children raised on animal-based fats already have abnormally high deposits of fat in their arteries—the very beginnings of future heart disease. Instead of potato chips, Snickers bars, and other processed, saturated yuck, give your kids healthy, naturally occurring polyunsaturated fats in the form of nuts, avocados, soybeans, and oatmeal.

For infants, PCRM recommends they remain on breast milk for at least six months (Dr. McDougall recommends two years). If breast feeding is not possible, commercial soy formulas fortified with vitamins and minerals are an excellent option. The animal-based proteins found in dairy-based formulas, especially those derived from cows' milk, sometimes do not agree with infants' fragile digestive systems. Dairy-based formulas have also been linked to allergies, ear infections, and, more seriously, juvenile diabetes. Remember that infants require special soy-milk formulas; typical milk alternatives found in grocery stores, while delicious and healthy for adults, are not adequate for infants.

After six months, when the high iron supply an infant is born with begins to diminish, you can then add iron-fortified infant cereal mixed with either breast milk or soy formula. At around eight months, try adding fruit, such as mashed bananas, peaches, avocados, and applesauce. You can also try adding cooked and mashed vegetables: sweet potatoes, green beans, peas, and carrots. By eight months, most infants can digest whole-grain crackers, breads, and dry cereals, and you can also try adding higher-protein foods such as tofu and mashed beans.

Remember that growing children and teens can handle high-calorie diets better than adults—they need energy to grow! Frequent snacks in addition to their three square meals are fine, but promote snacking on fruits, nuts, and nut butters, as well as whole-grain-based foods. Load them up on dark green vegetables, including broccoli, spinach, kale, collard greens, turnip greens, beet greens, mustard greens, bok choy, and Swiss chard. A consistent supply of protein is important, so steer your kids toward legumes, including pinto, black, and kidney beans; lentils; split peas; navy beans; and chickpeas. Most kids love hummus! Protein-rich soy products such as tofu, tempeh, edamame, and home-made veggie burgers are great as well.

Remember, this is one big plant-strong, lifelong adventure! You will be making changes—or introducing a lifestyle—that will have a lasting impact on your children. It's a gift that will keep on giving for years to come, and it all starts when you set a healthy example of what plant-strong living is all about!

Kole and Sophie

People always ask Jill and me how our children eat. So here's a brief history from Jill herself!

I breast-fed both kids as long as possible. I weaned Kole at fifteen months when I became pregnant with Sophie; then I nursed Sophie for a little more than two years.

When the kids were about eight months old, we started introducing solid foods: whole-grain cereals, mashed bananas, applesauce, avocado, lentil soup, mashed beans and bean broth, oatmeal, and sweet potatoes. I loved making homemade baby food, including pears and steamed kale blended with a little bit of cinnamon.

Similar to adults, every child's palate and digestive system is different. It is fair to say that Kole (who is five) is a picky eater, and Sophie (three) will eat almost anything, except when she is emulating her big brother! Therefore, I experimented with small amounts of spice—Kole tended to like his food plain, and Sophie spicy. We found that Kole had no problem with whole-grain cereals at eight months, but Sophie's little digestive system could not handle them: she became extremely constipated so we cut the grains altogether and focused her diet solely on fruits, legumes, and vegetables until she was slightly older than one year.

For allergy reasons, we were careful about not introducing nuts or berries until both of them turned two.

As the kids grew, we started talking to them about their diet. And once Kole started relating to the stories we were reading to him at bedtime, he became curious about animals as well—see chapter

33 for his reactions. The great thing is that everything we tell the kids is backed up by what they see in nature and the world around us, so it makes sense to them. I think it would be much more difficult to try to explain to our kids why we let other people kill the animals we love and then eat them.

And we kept the vegetables coming, and so should you! Human breast milk is sweet, which gives babies a natural propensity toward sweet foods. So fruits are an easy transition food as solids are being introduced. Babies will try anything, but when toddlerhood comes into full swing, many kids start shying away from anything that's not fruit or a carb. Keep giving them as many vegetables as possible!

Our kids also eat nuts and naturally fatty foods, such as avocado. Kids can, and should, eat more naturally fatty foods than adults. Their growing little bodies need it.

The most important lesson I have learned is to never give up. Kids go through phases, and so of course we too experience the "I don't like carrots!" dinner conversation (that of course occurs the day after they ate two huge carrots!). Just like all other aspects in parenting, just roll with it and don't give up. Our kids get at least one vegetable on their plates at both lunch and dinner. Keep dishing it out and don't be daunted by a phase.

Another tip is to "hide" some vegetables: soup is a great way to do this, and so are veggie burgers. I even put chickpeas in the chocolate chip cookies I make!

The last tip: if your child gets on a kick for one food, let them go!! Kole was on a carrot kick once— lunch, dinner, snack: carrots, carrots, carrots. And

(continued)

Sophie goes through phases when she can eat an entire large avocado in one sitting. Their little bodies know what they need, and when you are feeding them natural, whole foods you don't have to worry.

Finally, we know the plan is working, because both Kole and Sophie are healthy and happy kids!

26

Take Plants, Not Supplements

Ever taken a stroll down the health food aisle of your local supermarket or drugstore? You've probably seen the endless parade of vitamins and supplements as well as shakes, pills, powders, mixes, and more from ten thousand different brands. Some contain one vitamin, others lots of vitamins, and still others seem to be things you've never even heard of. But in the end, all those supplements seem to do the same darn thing—that is, offer you the chance to take in all your daily vitamins with one gulp.

Which are actually important? Which do you need to take?

Well, for you lucky plant munchers, the answer is simple: None of them! That's right. With a proper plant-strong diet, you don't have to worry about all those bulky, expensive pills and disgusting shakes. That's because all the essential vitamins and minerals you could ever want can be found in good old fruits, vegetables, whole grains, and legumes.

Our bodies were never meant to consume isolated vitamins in a con-centrated pill form. They were meant to consume whole foods so that all of the powerful vitamins, minerals, antioxidants, and fibers work as a team the way Mother Nature intended. In fact, several meta-analyses have shown the detrimental effects when antioxidants such as vitamin A, E, and selenium are taken in pill form—much to the dismay of many pill companies.

Let's break it down by discussing some of the most important vita-mins, starting with none other than the letter A. The type of vitamin A found in all plants is actually beta-carotene, which is the precursor to vitamin A.

Vitamin A is needed primarily by our eyes, especially for low-light vision. It also helps coat our retinas and mucous membranes, protecting them against infectious disease. Most supplements are chemically infused with vitamin A, but instead of popping pills it's far easier to get your daily vitamin A intake by eating vegetables. And one of my favorite veggies happens to be the reigning heavyweight vitamin-A champion of the world: carrots. One 7-inch, Bugs Bunny–style carrot is jam-packed with more than 200 percent of your daily vitamin A requirement. This is one of the main reasons Steve Austin, the "six million dollar man," had such good eyesight—he loved carrots!

Can't find a carrot? Well you're in luck: Vitamin A is also abundant in dark, leafy greens; yellow vegetables and fruits; broccoli, spinach, turnip greens, squash, sweet potatoes, pumpkins, cantaloupe, and apricots.

Now some of your meaty friends might bring up vitamin D—surely that's found only in animals? Nope. You can also find it in sunshine-grown mushrooms. That's right, the only plant food that has vitamin D is good old 'shrooms! And of course, you can find it in all of the fortified cereals and soy products. But unless you're a true troglodyte, you don't really have anything to worry about. Why? Because our bodies synthesize appropriate amounts of vitamin D naturally from as little as 15 to 20 minutes of sun exposure. So step outdoors and enjoy!

Probably the most common type of supplement you'll see is vitamin C tablets. These guys tend to be chewable, taste like candy, come in big plastic jugs, and, like other supplements, are probably not necessary. A long time ago, back when sailors would spend months and years at sea, vitamin C deficiency was a serious problem, leading to excruciating diseases like scurvy. When a daily ration of limes proved to solve the problem, the English sailors ate so much of these fruits they became known as limeys.

If you don't feel like puckering up for a lime or lemon, though, try guavas, papayas, strawberries, kiwis, cantaloupe, oranges, and grapefruit. Far more tasty than popping a pill.

At some point, one of your Paleo buddies is bound to start screaming about vitamin B12. Tell him or her to read chapter 4. But remember once again that humans require only trace amounts of this vitamin, and plant-superhero eaters have very low rates of B12 deficiency. In fact, more meat eaters have B12 deficiencies because of gastrointestinal and inadequate-absorption issues. You can get lots of B12 from fortified foods such as cereals and plant-based milks, or in Red Star nutritional yeast. But if you do decide to supplement with this one vitamin because you're not eating any of these foods, the good news is that there are no known toxic effects of excessive amounts of B12.

What about minerals? Do plants provide adequate amounts of zinc, iron, and magnesium? You betcha! Zinc is an essential one, which promotes healthy skin and immune systems and enhances cell reproduction and tissue growth. And lucky for you it's found in some pretty darn delicious plant-based foods. Lentils, beans, seeds, nuts, green vegetables, and whole grains are all adequate sources of zinc.

Now, lots of uninformed "meatsters" might try to convince you that plant-based iron is not as well absorbed as the iron found in a steak and can, therefore, lead to iron deficiency. Studies routinely prove that iron deficiency is no more common among plant-based eaters than among animal and dairy eaters. In fact, according to the USDA, the top sources of iron are from plants such as collard greens, lentils, and broccoli. Check out chapter 5 for more on iron.

One more mineral: magnesium. Magnesium deficiency is extremely rare—and even rarer among plant-chompers. That's because this deficiency is usually the result of excess consumption of other things, including fat and calcium, which can inhibit the absorption of magnesium. Well, rest assured! As you know by now, animal-based products and by-products are especially high in saturated fats and calcium—the perfect recipe for developing a magnesium deficiency!—while plants contain moderate, appropriate amounts of everything. For especially magnesium-rich foods, try almonds, avocados, bananas, whole grains, lentils, nuts, and seeds.

Let's not forget folate (vitamin B9), which many nutritionally challenged doctors will insist their patients take. The word *folate* is derived from the word *foliage* because the vitamin originates in root vegetables. Forage through the foliage section and get all the folate you need.

If you're eating a plant-sorry diet of potato chips, French fries, and dozens of diet sodas, then you won't be getting the right amount of the minerals and vitamins your body needs. But if you eat a plant-safe diet of whole grains and a variety of legumes, and peel your vitamins and minerals from fruits and vegetables, then you've got your game on! Now you'll be getting a cornucopia of vitamins and minerals in a whole package made by Mother Nature, not Nature's Mother, and you'll be as healthy as a Canadian moose.

27

Barbecue + Meat = Danger

I live in Texas. As far as we're concerned, there are few better things to do in this world than barbecue. Where else in the world do you find teams that actually compete in BBQ contests on the weekends?

But if you don't eat meat, "grilling" used to limit you to grazing on a hamburger bun with a slice of tomato, some iceberg lettuce, and a smear of ketchup. All of that has changed, thanks to two separate discoveries. First, people have realized that vegetables taste amazing when roasted over an open flame. Second, it turns out that there's a lot of research showing eating grilled meat can cause cancer.

That's right: When you grill any kind of meat, including chicken, beef, pork, and fish, what you are really doing is growing carcinogens on it. There are two that appear only in grilled meat: heterocyclic amines (HCAs) and polycyclic aromatic hydrocarbons (PAHs).

HCAs are what you get when the natural amino acids, sugars, and creatine in meat react at high temperatures. You know those tasty char marks that backyard barbecuers always try to get on their burgers and steaks? Those are really carcinogen marks, where all the HCAs accumulate.

PAHs are created when fat drips onto an open flame, causing a flash of fire and sizzle that sears the chemical into the surface of the meat, adding another layer of carcinogen. The longer and hotter you cook the meat, the more carcinogens you get. Boiling creates comparatively few PAHs, baking creates a few more, and grilling, with its high temperatures and long cooking times, practically breeds the nasty little things.

HCAs and PAHs are no joke: They're linked to higher rates of colorectal, pancreatic, breast, and prostate cancer. PAHs are linked to stomach cancer. A recent analysis of thirty separate studies found that 80 percent showed a strong correlation between consumption of well-done meat and cancer in different areas of the body.

According to the scientists who study HCAs, the five worst meats to grill, in order from bad to the drop-dead worst, are: hamburger, salmon, pork, steak, and the humble chicken breast. Even without the skin, chicken produces almost twice the level of HCAs as steak and over one hundred times that of hamburger!

Plants aren't on that list because they don't contain the raw materials for HCAs. Creatine, one of the carcinogen's key ingredients, isn't found in plants no matter how much you burn them, so the HCA-producing chemical reactions can't take place. Plants also contain cancer-fighting agents like carotenoids and beta-carotene.

But don't grill just any vegetable. If you've ever eaten one of those generic grilled veggie plates served at a lot of restaurants, you know that not all plants are even made for the flames. For the best grilling, first choose plants that contain a lot of water so they won't dry out. Most veggies have a high liquid content, but you'll want to avoid carrots and potatoes because they do more shriveling than actual cooking on the grill unless you wrap them in a bit of foil.

Next, choose plants whose bold flavors will complement the smoky goodness of the open flames: bell peppers, corn on the cob, onions, squash, mushrooms, and pineapple are among my favorites.

Finally, have some non-oil salad dressing or marinade on hand to keep your veggies moist if they start looking a little parched. "Grilled" shouldn't mean "withered."

Don't forget about the fungi and the grains either. Mushrooms sizzle like few other foods. A good portobello mushroom brushed with barbecue sauce, a pinch of salt, and plenty of black pepper makes one heck of a great "burger." Also, a simple dough of whole wheat flour, salt, water, and yeast, like the recipe for Jill's Maple Whole Wheat Bread Dough on page 164, can be grilled to make an awesome flatbread.

Remember, just because veggies contain no HCAs and non-cancer-causing levels of PAHs doesn't mean you should eat nothing but grilled veggies. When you put any food over an open flame, it soaks up carcinogens that may be present in charcoal, propane, and/or lighter fluid. Ovens and stoves were invented for a reason.

Of course, carnivores offer a slew of feeble solutions to the whole "eating grilled meat gives you cancer" problem: Cook your meat in the microwave before finishing it on the grill, use lots of marinade, or—my personal favorite—don't char your meat. If you don't char, you may as well not barbecue.

We've made entire salads at the firehouse with grilled vegetables, and managed to get perfect char marks on everything: tomatoes, potatoes, bell peppers, carrots, yellow squash, mushrooms, even the romaine lettuce! The recipes on pages 180 and 240 are specifically made for the grill.

I don't know about you, but I like to have my tofu and eat it too. That's why I grill veggies—all char, no carcinogens.

28

Oil Is the New Snake Oil

Study after study after study has proven the benefits of eating more fruits and vegetables, and every day more and more people are adding them to their diet. Unfortunately, lots of food companies are taking advantage of these healthy decisions by pedaling alleged plant-based products that claim to offer the same benefits as real plants.

For the grand Poobah of deceptive advertising, look no further than public enemy number 1: vegetable oil.

Now, vegetable oil may sound as though it's good for you. After all, it has the word "vegetable" in it, and the container says "heart healthy." Not only that, everyone is always saying how good olive oil is for you.

Well, like many lies, this fallacy ultimately boils down to money. Back in the 1950s, the seed oil industry found itself in crisis mode after traditional paint and plastic production switched to cheaper petroleum-based sources. In desperate need of a new market, seed oil producers began touting the "heart protective" benefits of vegetable oils. The "lipid hypothesis," as it became known, argued that polyunsaturated fats in the blood helped reduce cholesterol levels.

Until now, the lipid hypothesis enjoyed widespread consensus, even though the science backing it was suspect. (Some of the rather dubious early experiments involved rabbits and a Russian researcher who never conducted any clinical trials with humans.) But the truth is that while moderate, natural amounts of polyunsaturated fats found in nuts and other whole foods *do* promote heart health, the processed oils derived from them most certainly *do not*.

Now the more astute of your oil-guzzlin' friends may, like mine, say something like: "Hey, Rip, vegetable oil is liquid, so that means it's unsaturated fat, which is found in nuts and other good things." Well they're right—sort of. Moderate amounts of unsaturated fats can be found in olives, peanuts, avocados, and many more excellent plant-based products. But imagine taking a million olives, peanuts, and avocados and then squeezing and chemically processing the heck out of them until all that's left is a plastic jug full of liquid fat.

Vegetable oil manufacturers would like you to think that this freak-ish chemical concoction is healthy and great for cooking. But here's what they don't tell you: The manufacturers add hydrogen atoms to a liquid veggie oil under heat and pressure to "hydrogenate" it. These oils are then more stable and can be used in high-heat situations. This increases the shelf life of the products, but it doesn't increase your shelf life—these man-made fats have no health benefits, raise total cho-lesterol, and contribute to coronary artery disease.

You may know another Frankenstein fat: trans fat, aka trans-fatty acids. They are a by-product of the hydrogenation process. Trans fat increases the risk of heart disease. You'll often see food packaging saying "no trans fat," and many cities have banned the use of these in restaurants, with good reason—they increase total cholesterol levels and LDL, aka lethal-cholesterol levels; they reduce HDL, aka healthy-cholesterol levels; and they even seem to interfere with the body's optimum use of omega-3 fatty acids.

But what about at restaurants, you ask? What about all that lovely olive oil that I dip my healthy, whole-grain bread into? I'm not cooking with it, so I don't have to worry about the whole trans fat business, right?

Unfortunately, the truth is that all oils—cooked and uncooked—are unhealthy. As I said, oils are simply liquid fat. A long time ago, in a galaxy far, far, away, they may have been part of delicious vegetables or nuts, but to get into their current bottled form they've had to be end-lessly squeezed and extracted and processed until they bear no resem-blance to their former selves.

If you've ever put some leftovers in the fridge, you've probably noticed that the next day they have a slightly stale taste. You see, vegeta-ble oils are composed of long-chain fatty acids that are highly unstable. Even if refrigerated for only a few hours, such oils can rapidly oxidize and turn rancid. When mixed with your stomach's digestive enzymes, these polyunsaturated oils decompose into a toxic, trans-fatty cocktail that wreaks havoc on your body.

As noted physiologist Dr. Ray Peat notes: "All oils, even if they're organic, cold-pressed, unprocessed, bottled in glass, and stored away from heat and light, are damaging. These oils have no shelf life at all…and when they're warmed to body temperature, they disintegrate even faster. Once ingested, they bind with cells and interfere with every chemical reaction in the body. The results are hormone imbalances, inflammation, and all kinds of illness."

Sound bad? Well look at this: In 2000, Dr. Robert Vogel of the University of Maryland conducted a study in which he measured otherwise healthy participants' arterial blood flow before and after consumption of olive oil and bread. Afterward, Dr. Vogel determined that olive oil had constricted blood flow in the subjects' vessels by 31 percent! He discovered that oils damage the fragile endothelial lining in our blood vessels by causing arteries to constrict, promoting the buildup of plaque.

Then there's the so-called latest and greatest of all the hot new oils, coconut oil. Specifically, people are hooting and hollering about the healthy medium-chain triglycerides (MCTs) that supposedly make coconut oil and its accompanying coconut products superfoods. Stop the presses! The reality is that coconut oil is 92 percent saturated fat (see chart below)! About 65 percent of that comes from MCTs, but the rest comes from LCTs (long-chain triglycerides), the same type of artery-clogging, cancer-promoting, and diabetes-enhancing saturated fats that are in red meat, chicken, and pork.

Nutrition Facts

Serving Size 13 g

Amount Per Serving

Calories 116	Calories from Fat 116

	% Daily Value*
Total Fat 14g	21%
Saturated Fat 12g	58%
Trans Fat	
Cholesterol 0mg	0%
Sodium 0mg	0%
Total Carbohydrade 0g	0%
Dietary Fiber 0g	0%
Sugars 0g	
Protein 0g	

Vitamin A	0% •	Vitamin C	0%
Calcium	0% •	Iron	0%

*Percent Daily Values are based on a 2,000 calorie diet. Your daily values may be higher or lower depending on your calorie needs.

NutritionData.com

One tablespoon of coconut oil

So instead of getting your fat from an extracted third-class poser, why not get it from whole-food sources that offer all of the good falsely associated with oils and none of the bad: olives, oats, leafy greens (9 to 11 percent fat), fruit (yes, even fruit has fat), whole grains, legumes, nuts, and seeds.

My father, Dr. Caldwell Esselstyn Jr., likes to tell a story about his good friend Reverend William Valentine, who, in 1990, underwent quintuple bypass surgery. After the procedure, the good reverend adhered to a strict plant-based diet, during which his weight dropped from 210 to 156 pounds. But after fourteen healthy, plant-based years, Reverend Valentine developed a recurrence of angina. After assuring my father that he ate only whole grains, fruit, vegetables, and legumes, he also mentioned the ample amounts of "heart-healthy" olive oil he'd started to consume with most meals. My father immediately instructed his friend to cut out the olive oil. Within two months, the reverend was angina-free and praising whole plants and the Lord!

OO

Let's take a closer look at the darling of all oils in America, our beloved olive oil (OO). Hold on to your britches! It takes about 1,375 squeezed olives to fill up a 32-ounce container of OO. OO is 100 percent fat, and at almost 120 calories per tablespoon, it is more calorie dense than any other food on the planet. It also has more empty calories than white flour or white sugar, is 14.5 percent saturated fat, and contains almost no vitamins or minerals. (It does have trace amounts of vitamin E and K, in percentages so small that if you wanted to get your daily supply of omega-3 fatty acids from OO, you'd have to chugalug about a half-pound bottle, or about 2,000 calories' worth.) Yowsie!

Here's the oily bottom line: Most Americans are downing 3 to 5 tablespoons a day (i.e., 360 to 600 empty calories) by dipping their bread into it, baking with it, drizzling it over salads, pouring it into stir-fries, and taking straight shots of it! Americans mistakenly think OO is magically reversing the ill effects of all the bad foods they've been shoveling down their throats. The sobering reality: OO is only contributing to Americans' heart disease and ever-increasing waistlines. OO stands for zero and zilch of anything good!

Nutrition Facts

Serving Size 13 g

Amount Per Serving	
Calories 119	Calories from Fat 119

	% Daily Value*
Total Fat 14g	21%
Saturated Fat 2g	9%
Trans Fat	
Cholesterol 0mg	0%
Sodium 0mg	0%
Total Carbohydrade 0g	0%
Dietary Fiber 0g	0%
Sugars 0g	
Protein 0g	

Vitamin A	0%	Vitamin C	0%
Calcium	0%	Iron	0%

*Percent Daily Values are based on a 2,000 calorie diet. Your daily values may be higher or lower depending on your calorie needs.

NutritionData.com

29

There's Something
Fishy About Fish Oil

We've all been hearing a lot about fish oil recently. This stuff can do everything! It's the best thing since sliced bread! It's better than vitamins and minerals! It keeps you heart healthy! It keeps your mind strong! It wards off Alzheimer's, Parkinson's, and depression. And more!

But is fish oil really snake oil in disguise?

The active ingredients in fish oil are omega-3 fatty acids. Omega-3s are essential to your body. And sure, fish oil contains a lot of omega-3s, but, like so many animal products, it also has a lot of other terrible stuff that's bad for you—and bad for the environment.

The first problem with fish oil is that it's made from juicing the discarded parts of fish. According to a 2009 *New York Times* article, a lot of American fish oils come from menhaden, a member of the herring family that not only cleans the oceans through filter feeding, but is also the basis for the entire food chain in the Atlantic Ocean. Too bad for the sea: Menhaden are going the way of the dodo due to their usefulness to humans. (Besides health supplements, manufacturers use them for fertilizer, lipstick, salmon feed, and paint.)

Even if you can stomach the idea of swallowing a pill filled with a paint ingredient, you should still prepare yourself for some nasty side effects. The least harmful is the "fish burp" that is exactly what it sounds like. Raw fish oils tend to irritate the stomach, and can cause indigestion, nausea, diarrhea, and fish farts that will peel the paint off the walls of your home!

Menhaden-flavored gasses might be the least of your gastric worries, but that doesn't make them any nicer. More expensive brands of fish oil claim to be odorless and tasteless when you belch them back up, but even their fans admit that the pills give them gastric fish reminders throughout the day. Their friends notice it too: Oil pill poppers often have fishy breath and toots.

Worse, fish oil can thin your blood. It's not a problem for everyone, but people who are already on blood thinners can get nosebleeds and blood in their urine, and even suffer strokes from bleeding in the brain. People who already have bleeding problems, such as ulcers, and those taking cocktails of medications are particularly at risk.

Toxic chemicals in the ocean bio-accumulate in fish oil the same way that toxicants in the air and ground accumulate in cow fat. Many pill heads don't realize that even though they aren't actually eating fish, they're still ingesting all of the contaminants in the fish's flesh. A 2010 study found that some fish oil pills contain high levels of toxicants such as PCBs because the fish they are made from absorb the carcinogens from the foods they eat. Of the estimated 200 brands of fish oil pills on the market, the Mateel Environmental Justice Foundation tested ten and found that all contained some levels of toxic chemicals, with three actually exceeding the government's daily limit for carcinogen exposure.

So far, I've covered problems with fresh fish oil, but unless you are making your own pills, even freshness isn't guaranteed. You won't smell or taste anything funny, aside from the fish burps, but some fish oil pills also contain oxidative by-products. Translation: They're rancid. Fish oil starts to go rancid, or to oxidate, as soon as it comes out of the fish. It continues breaking down inside the pill until you swallow it. Although many companies claim that their pills are good for years, the data show something different. Scientists link oxidative by-products to heart disease, so instead of helping your heart, rancid fish oil might actually hurt it in the long run.

As you can see, the risks of this animal product outweigh its benefits. Besides, you don't need to eat fish or take fish oil in order to get omega-3s; you just have to know which plants offer it. The most accessible of these are nuts and seeds. Ground flaxseeds, chia seeds, and English walnuts all have plenty of the essential fatty acids. Beans and leafy greens are another excellent source. Kale, leeks, broccoli, lima beans, and soybeans all are convenient and easy to fit into meals. Seaweeds, such as the Japanese wakame and nori (the black stuff around the outside of a sushi roll) as well as our American spirulina, also contain omega-3s but are harder to find—look for them in health food stores or Asian specialty shops.

The omega-3 all-star is flaxseed. Don't be intimidated because you don't know how to eat it; these little seeds have been considered a health food by just about every civilized culture since the ancient Egyptians—and they pack more omega-3s than any other plant source. Buy preground seeds or grind them yourself, then sprinkle them over your favorite foods by the teaspoonful. (Note: Grinding is a must; otherwise, the omega-3s aren't as bio-available—they will just pass through your system.)

I put flaxseeds in my Rip's Big Bowl cereal and homemade salad dressings, stir it into pasta sauces, bake it into bread, and sometimes just snack on the seeds, like Roman gladiators used to. Another omega-3 all-star that can be used just like ground flaxseed, but doesn't have to be ground for bio-availability, is chia seeds—yes, those little seeds you can use to grow funny-looking creature pets with green hair, or you can eat to get omega-3 fats!

30

Poops from Heaven

The other day I was talking to Lydia, a lovely woman who had just attended one of my presentations. Lydia is slightly overweight. She also mentioned that her cholesterol level was way too high, her HDL (her healthy cholesterol) was too low, and her LDL (her lethal cholesterol) was off the charts. Plus, she had just been diagnosed as prediabetic. And so she knew that she was the perfect candidate for going on a plant-based diet. She was jazzed and ready to take her health to the next level.

Except for one thing—Lydia was worried about the bathroom. Not the actual bathroom, that is. She was afraid that if she stopped eating meat and eggs, she'd be going to the toilet all the time.

The odd fact is that a lot of people worry that a plant-based diet will make them use the bathroom more. Listen to me! Damn straight it will! And that's a good thing.

Here's why: The National Institute of Diabetes and Digestive and Kidney Diseases (NIDDK) reports that constipation is one of the most common gastrointestinal problems in the United States: More than four million people report frequent cases of it each year.

Although constipation is technically defined as having fewer than three bowel movements a week, everyone is different and there is no absolute number of number twos that people have to miss before they are considered constipated—and certainly not before they *feel* constipated.

If you are having fewer than normal bowel movements—and if, when you do have them, getting that crap out of your system feels like a lot of work—chances are that you are another of the millions of constipated people. Women and the elderly suffer from this problem more often than anyone else—or at least they report it more. Many other millions are estimated to suffer from it too, but they are either overly embarrassed to talk about their condition with a doctor, or simply are so used to it that they don't think this kind of pain is out of the ordinary.

So don't worry—you're not alone! People of all ages, races, and genders have trouble on the toilet seat. For many it is simply uncomfortable and embarrassing, but constipation can also lead to hemorrhoids, anal fissures (essentially tears in the skin around the anus), anal prolapse (where some of your intestinal lining leaks out of your body), and fecal impactions, in which so much waste builds up in your colon that you are unable to pass it. By that point a bit of embarrassment is not the first thing on your mind. Pain is.

In fact, a woman at one of my speeches told me she had been to the bathroom just *once* in the last month, and her poor mother, who hadn't been to the bathroom in over a month, had just had surgery to remove impacted feces. That is really, really sad. Especially because it is so completely unnecessary!

The NIDDK estimates that Americans spend $725 million every year on laxatives. That's like taking the GDP of the West African country Guinea-Bissau and flushing it down the toilet.

The number is even crazier considering that constipation isn't actually a disease. It's a symptom of a bad diet. What's the number one cause of constipation in America? A diet containing too much fat, meat, eggs, dairy, and refined foods, and not enough fiber. There is zero fiber in meat and dairy products. Fiber can only be found in plants—nature's laxative!

To understand how these foods affect your digestive system, let's take a fantastic voyage down to the inner reaches of your colon. If you stretched yours out to its full length, it would reach about five feet. This long organ moves food from one end to the other through a process called peristalsis.

If you imagine squeezing the last of the toothpaste from the tube, you'll have a fair idea of how peristalsis works. Along the way, the colon sucks water out of the food and turns it into waste, aka poop. If the colon is slow, or if it absorbs too much water, the waste gets dry and hard, making it difficult to pass. (Imagine trying to work a bowl of dry corn flakes out of your toothpaste tube.)

Meat is especially hard to digest. It contains zero fiber and the protein-dense animal muscle in it requires your stomach to secrete more acid and your pancreas to secrete more enzymes just to get it through. Our digestive systems aren't made for this kind of hard work. You might remember from chapter 7 that carnivores have short, highly acidic digestive systems that move meat through quickly so it doesn't putrefy. Your colon takes about eighteen to thirty-six hours to move food from one end to the other. That's a lot of strain on your digestive system.

When it comes to digestion, the real benefit of plant foods is their bulk, water, and fiber. The real problem with animal foods is their lack of fiber. Fiber and water create bulky stools that push out on the colon and cause peristalsis, which means the colon then contracts, pushing the stool forward. That's the pattern: expand, contract, move. Without the fiber and water to create bulk, stools are hard and small and don't facilitate peristalsis—and so we must sit there pushing and squeezing to get them to move.

Of course, the easiest way to keep your waste soft and your colon happy is to eat plenty of fruits, vegetables, beans, and whole grains, which, as we've discussed, are the source of the magic ingredient fiber. The term "fiber" is just a catchall name for the parts of these plants that your body can't digest.

There are two types of fiber, soluble and insoluble. Soluble fiber gets its name because it dissolves in water. It's found in plants such as oats, nuts, beans, barley, flax, carrots, apples, and oranges. In your lower intestine, it has a gel-like consistency that slides right through you. Nice! Insoluble fiber doesn't dissolve and moves through you basically unchanged. It's in leafy greens, root veggies, and whole-grain products.

The American Dietetic Association recommends that people eat around 20 to 35 grams of fiber a day. Guess how much most Americans eat? A measly 5 to 14 grams. Guess how much a plant-strong eating machine like me enjoys each day? A powerful 50 to 75 grams! In fact, the Rip's Big Bowl recipe is loaded with 40 grams of protein and close to 40 grams of fiber! It's a veritable fiber Whopper! And as you can imagine, I'm as regular as a Swiss commuter train. I can't remember the last time I was logjammed. It's a real joy to have quick, easy, and gratifying poops. No doubt about it.

Speaking of quick, my brother-in-law, who is also plant-strong, was remarking how his speedy dumps are a nuisance. He'll take along a book or magazine to read in the men's library, but after 45 to 60 seconds—the time it takes him to complete a successful download—he's wondering why he bothered to bring reading materials at all. The truth is that once you become plant powered, your dumps will take as long as your pees.

So I'll tell you just what I told Lydia: Fiber will not give you diarrhea. Ever. One of the worst fiber myths is that it's edible Liquid Plumr. In general, fiber will simply help normalize the whole elimination process. Don't think of fiber as something that will make you go to the bathroom uncontrollably; think of it as something that will smooth out your digestion and keep food flowing the way it should, neither too fast nor too slow.

Go plant-strong. It will be a moving experience!

31

Carbs Are King!

You may have tried some of the trendy, low-carb diets that have been making the rounds in recent years. Unfortunately, Atkins and other supposedly well-researched diets have reinforced the misconception that carbohydrates are somehow bad for you, and succeeded in making the vast majority of America carbophobic.

Stop being a carb scaredy-cat and start enjoying unrefined carbohydrates as part of a healthy and satisfying plant-strong diet! Carbohydrates are our number one energy source, so don't even think about giving them up.

The problem is that the low-carb/high-protein diets give all carbohydrates—including whole grains, beans, vegetables, and even fruit—a bad name. I am in complete agreement with those in the high-protein camp who say refined carbohydrates are the worst: Soda pop, donuts, candy bars, fruit juice, white pasta, white rice, white bread, and fried chips all are filled with empty calories and have been stripped of their fiber, water, vitamins, minerals, and phytonutrients; they're a dangerous black hole of empty calories and nothing but Trouble with a capital T.

But good carbs are a must in creating a healthy you. Let's see why.

As I mentioned earlier, three macronutrients account for the calories in our diet: carbs, fat, and protein. Carbs are the largest and most important source. They help regulate our heart rate, our digestive system, and our breathing.

Here's the deal: *Processed* and *refined* carbs, like the junk found in packaged foods and fast-food meals, can make you fat. These bad boys typically lack any fiber, nutrients, or much of anything useful and are very concentrated in calories. But folks like Dr. Atkins have spread the misconception that *all* carbohydrates are alike.

Wrong!

The truth is that the majority of your calories should come from unrefined, unprocessed complex carbs and simple carbs found in fruits, veggies, and whole grains. These excellent carbs are converted into glucose, which is basically gasoline for our bodies.

Processed carbs, on the other hand, have been chemically altered by humans. These "Frankencarbs," stripped of all fiber and minerals and vitamins, are rich in calories and digested more quickly by the body, and can cause your blood sugar levels to spike. This, in turn, shoves your pancreas into insulin-pumping overdrive, inundating blood cells with extra glucose at pendulum-like intervals and leaving you fatigued and even more hungry. Why wouldn't you be? Most nutrients, fiber, and water have been removed, so they don't fill you up and people often overeat. If you've ever had a bad case of the munchies, you probably know exactly what I'm talking about.

But hey, how the heck do I know which carbs are processed and which aren't? Well, if they're in a box full of fancy marketing, most likely they're processed. If you order them on a microphone from your car, they're probably processed. Processed carbs are shells of their former selves, and really shouldn't even be called carbohydrates.

But until the FDA gets its act together and requires packaging to label them as *Frankencarbs*, you'll need to be careful when looking for the real stuff. Whole and unprocessed carbs (both simple and complex) are abundant in a plant-based diet. They're found in vegetables; whole grains and whole-grain breads, pasta, and dry cereals; peas; beans; sweet potatoes; oats; brown rice; and fruit.

Unlike processed and refined Frankencarbs, whole-grain carbohydrates cause a slow and stable release of sugar into the bloodstream, which is then converted into energy by your body, rather than stored as fat. And because these natural carbohydrates retain all their water and energy, your stomach fills up fast, ensuring that you'll never overeat.

So drop the white bread for whole-grain bread, park the candy for fruit, ditch the soda pop for water, and bury the white pasta for whole-grain pasta. It'll make a world of difference, and you can stop being a carbophobe!

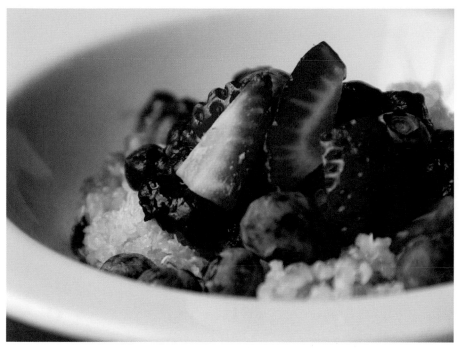

The Machu Picchu. *Photograph by Natala Constantine.*

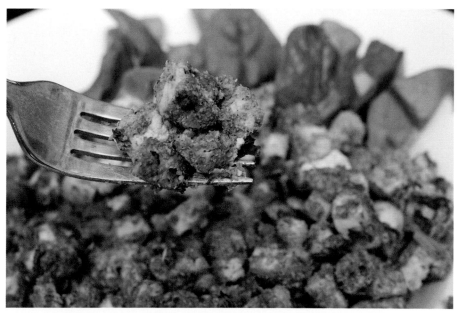

The Bouldin Creek Spicy Scrambler. *Photograph by Jane Esselstyn.*

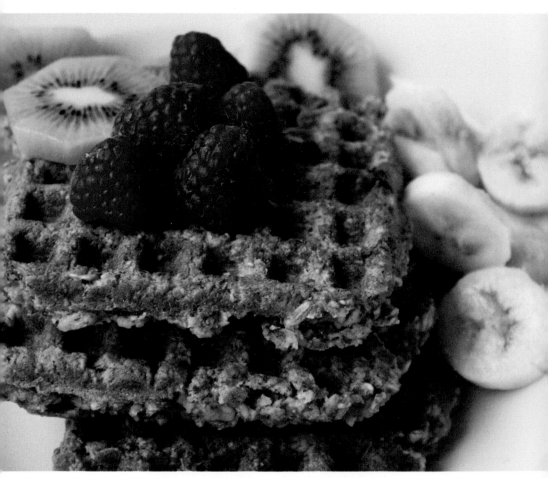

Zeb's Waffles. *Photograph by Jane Esselstyn.*

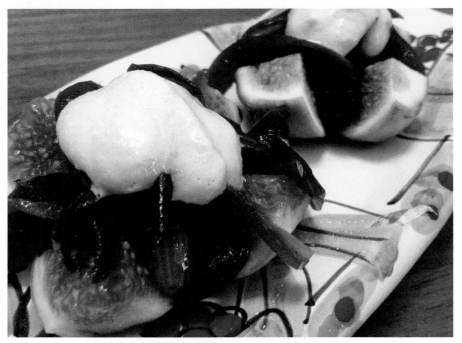

Split Figs with Cashew Cream and Caramelized Onions.
Photograph by Jane Esselstyn.

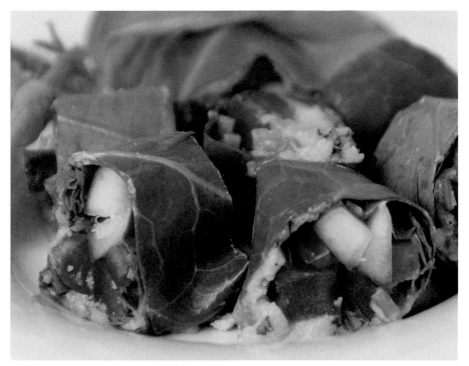

ACE's Original Hummus-Collard Wraps. *Photograph by Natala Constantine.*

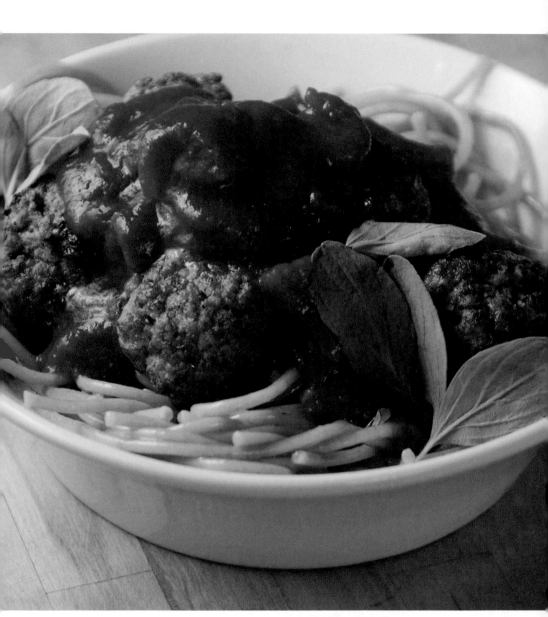

Spicy Italian Eat Balls. *Photograph by Matthew Constantine.*

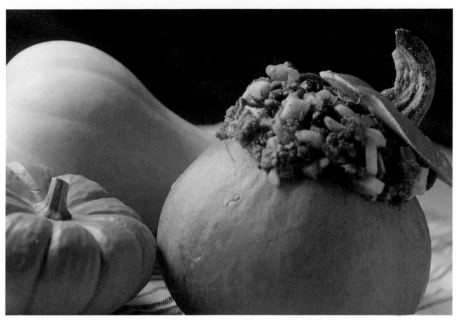

Fire Brigade Stuffing. *Photograph by Matthew Constantine.*

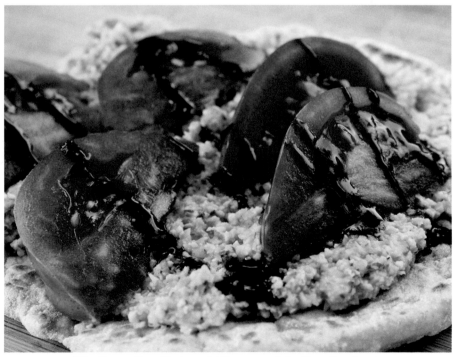

The Sunny Day Flatbread. *Photograph by Jane Esselstyn.*

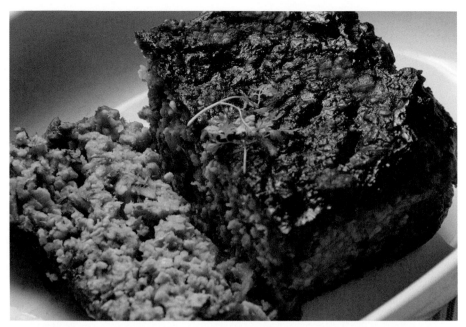

BBQ LOL (Lentil Oat Loaf). *Photograph by Matthew Constantine.*

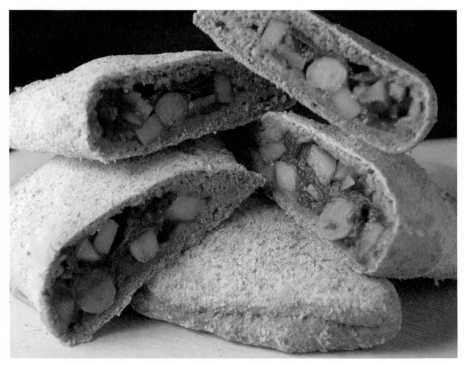

Village Potato Pockets. *Photograph by Matthew Constantine.*

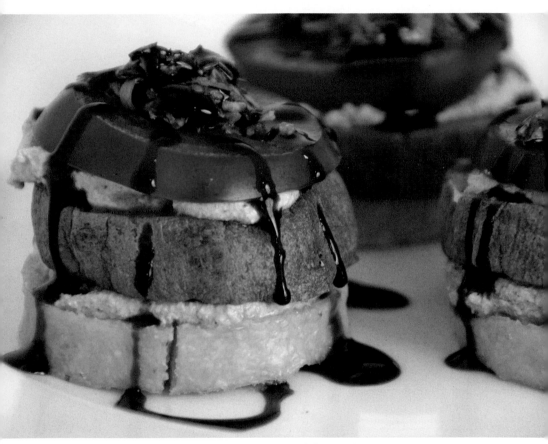

Dr. Seuss Stacked Polenta. *Photograph by Natala Constantine.*

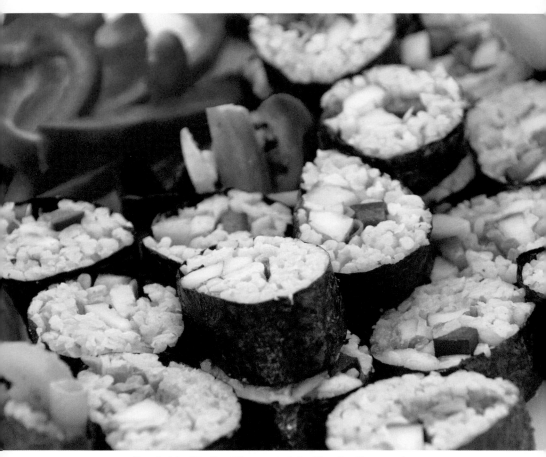

Jane's Nori Rolls. *Photograph by Natala Constantine.*

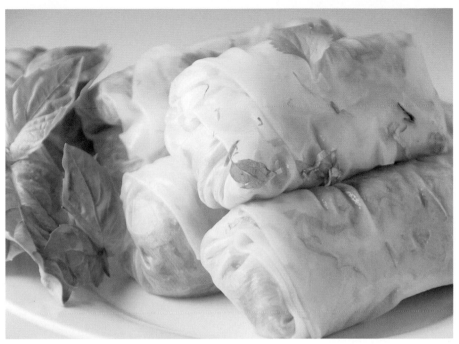

Toby's Thai Spring Rolls. *Photograph by Matthew Constantine.*

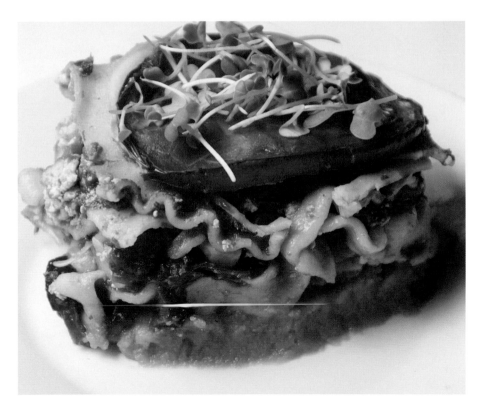

Raise-the-Barn Butternut Squash–Vegetable Lasagna.
Photograph by Matthew Constantine.

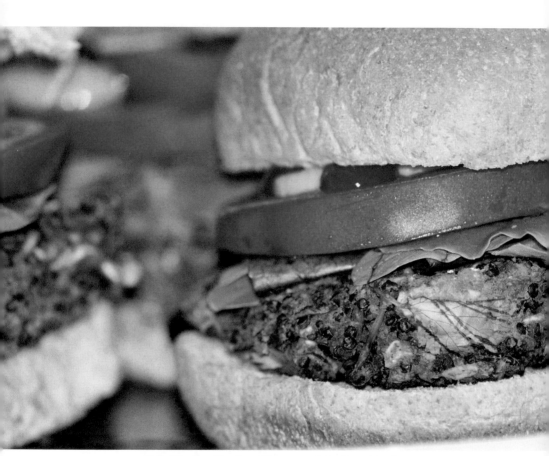

P.S. Chorizo Patties. *Photograph by Jane Esselstyn.*

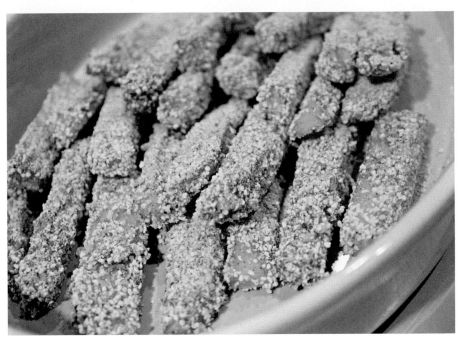

Crispy Polenta Strips. *Photograph by Jane Esselstyn.*

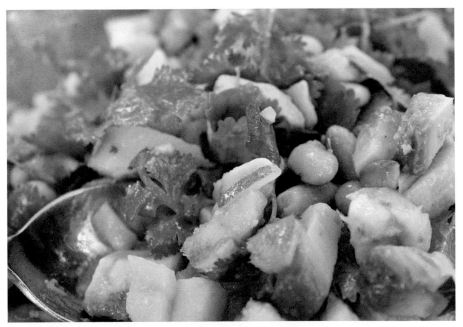

Fresh Anaheim and Edamame Spread. *Photograph by Jane Esselstyn.*

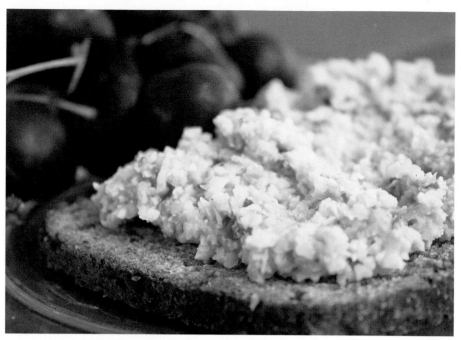

Lime-Mango Bean Salad. *Photograph by Jane Esselstyn.*

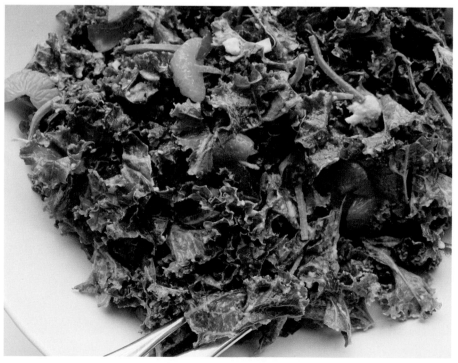

Kale Ceviche Salad. *Photograph by Jane Esselstyn.*

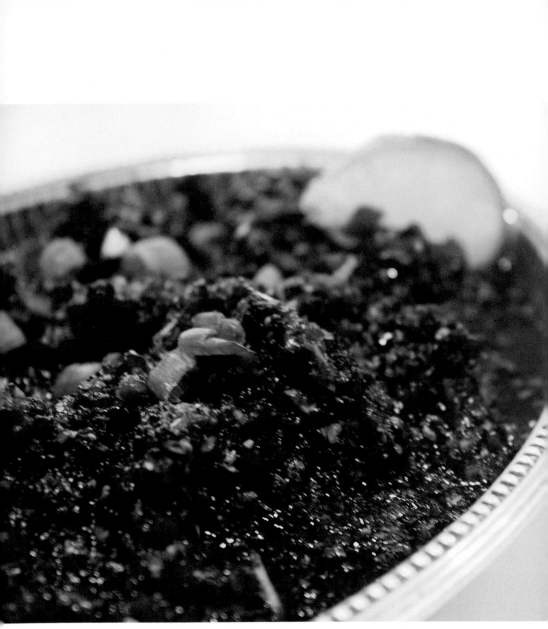

Down Under Cranberry Salsa. *Photograph by Jane Esselstyn.*

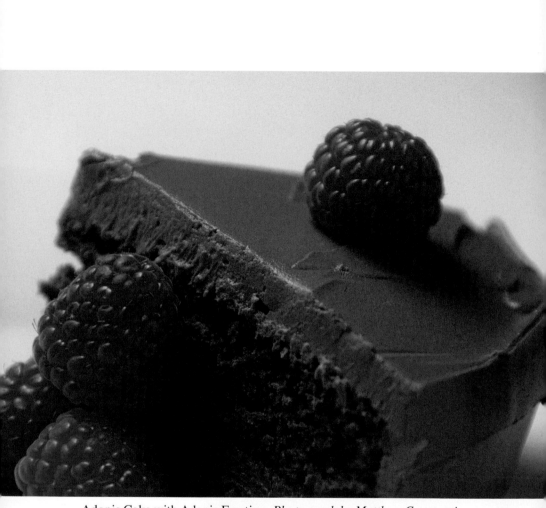

Adonis Cake with Adonis Frosting. *Photograph by Matthew Constantine.*

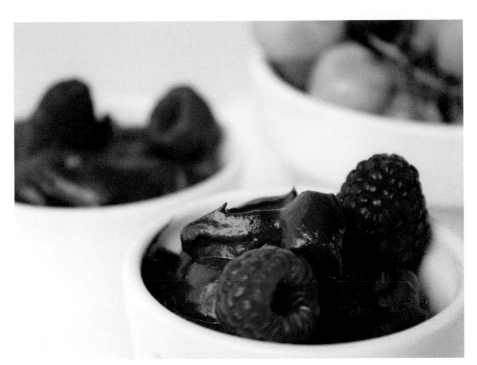

Chocomole. *Photograph by Crile Hart.*

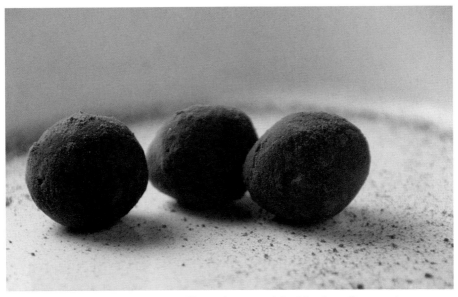

Bittersweet Chocolate Truffles. *Photograph by Matthew Constantine.*

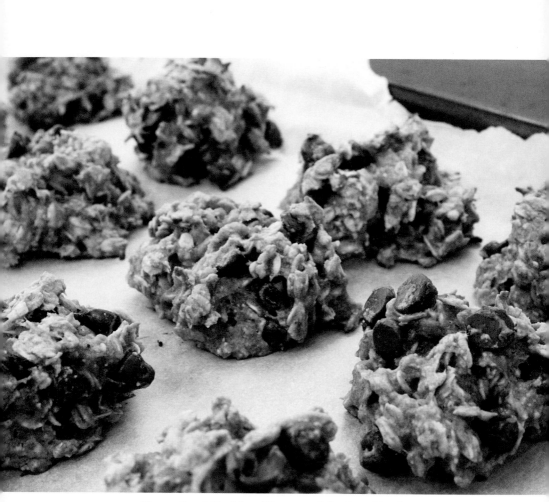

Damn Good Cookies. *Photograph by Jane Esselstyn.*

Juice Isn't the Way

If you want to be healthy, it isn't always enough to eat plant-based foods. It's possible, for instance, to carve out a plant-based diet that's composed of poor choices such as potato chips, pretzels, candy, and fruit juice.

Did I just say fruit juice? Healthy, vitamin-C-filled, all-natural fruit juice? The beverage we've been encouraging our kids to drink for decades?

Yes, I did. A glass of juice might not be as beneficial as you think. In fact, it could be harmful; new research says fruit juice contains so much sugar it can actually increase, rather than prevent, the risk of certain cancers. When I was a firefighter and we responded to medical emergency calls for diabetic patients with low blood sugar, the first thing we would give them to raise their glucose levels was orange juice. Believe it or not, a glass of OJ contains more sugar than a soda pop!

Not only that, because you seldom drink the freshly squeezed juice of a fruit but typically down only the processed and packaged liquid version of that fruit, you are missing many of the ingredients in fruit that protect against disease. In fact, in a 2011 Australian study published in the *Journal of the American Dietetic Association*, researchers found that eating apples, sprouts, cauliflower, or broccoli on a daily basis reduced the likelihood of rectal cancer, whereas three glasses of fruit juice a day increased the risk.

Scientists believe the high sugar content in juice may be the culprit (as a 2011 British study found), pointing out that many of the healthy benefits of fruit, such as fiber, vitamin C, and antioxidants, are lost during the

(continued)

juice's processing. In addition, when you separate fructose from the fiber (like you do when you whiz something up in a blender), you're getting a concentrated and pulverized form of fruit that bypasses your salivary digestive enzymes and causes a huge sugar spike, followed by an insulin spike, and then, believe it or not, about 30 percent of the fructose is converted straight to fat! So eat the fruit and get happily filled up with all the bulk, water, and fiber.

32

Don't Believe Everything
You Read About Soy

There's been a lot of talk about soy recently and it's all over the map: Soy is a miracle food; soy is bad for you. Soy is full of healthy phytochemicals; soy will make men grow breasts. Soy will keep you from getting cancer; soy will give you cancer. The truth is that a diet consisting solely or even mainly of soy is not a good idea. The best diet is one composed of many different foods. Eaten intelligently, however, soy is a terrific source of protein and a rich source of carbs, minerals, and essential fatty acids.

Although it's relatively new to the American diet, soy has been around longer than most foods we know. It comes from a bean that is native to East Asia and was first cultivated in China more than 1,300 years ago. Back then, soy was eaten fermented, cultured, and ground into a liquid that we now call soy milk.

In 1765 colonists brought the beans with them to the United States. But soybeans, which were used mostly as animal feed, didn't catch on as a crop in America until the early 1900s, when chemist George Washington Carver realized their nutritional benefits and discovered their ability to replenish nitrogen and minerals in soil. Based on his findings, Carver developed the first system of crop rotation in the United States. By 2007, soybeans had become a $27 billion industry, covering 22 percent of America's croplands, or 64.7 million acres.

The misconceptions about soy started when tofu was "discovered" by proponents—and manufacturers—of health foods in the 1990s, who then rushed to pin as many miraculous properties on it as possible: Soy lowers your cholesterol, soy protects against breast cancer, soy makes you smarter...yada, yada, yada. Unfortunately, some of these claims were often based only on scant preliminary evidence rather than robust long-term research. Longer studies and meta-analyses have since shown that eating soy won't make you immortal after all.

The most famous case of overstated findings was a study declaring that soy *will* reduce your LDL, or bad cholesterol. But you'd have to wolf down 50 grams of soy protein a day, or 1.5 pounds of tofu, just in case you were considering it.

On the other hand, the pet cause of a few anti-soy organizations has been to convince people that soy is more harmful than nuclear waste. These groups have accused soy of causing everything from cancer to brain atrophy. Their so-called evidence is usually based on partial readings of much more complex studies. They also love to crib quotes from research abstracts the way commercials for bad movies pull the few good lines out of really bad reviews.

The good news: There is credible scientific evidence that eating reasonable amounts of soy in a natural form won't do anything but fill you up and give you a lot of great nutrients.

And all those soy allergies you keep hearing about? Infants are the most common sufferers, but they usually grow out of them (unlike peanut allergies). Adults rarely have them at all.

There's a right way and a wrong way to eat soy, though. Asians generally eat it the right way: in its natural form, without additives and preservatives. Americans tend to eat it the wrong way—processed to death or pounded and ground into supplements. Some soy burgers contain more sodium than a grilled steak, and taking straight doses of soy protein, as some people do in their smoothies, hasn't been proven effective or even safe.

In addition, you'll find soy protein isolates as an ingredient (which most of the time are hexane-extracted) in most soy burgers, soy dogs, soy cheese, soy ice cream, and soy nuggets. This is a concentrated dose of isolated soy protein that has mega amounts of IGF-1, which is highly unhealthy and a tumor and cancer promoter.

In all the discussions of soy pros and cons, isoflavones are the questionable components. They are organic compounds that many people consider an invaluable health aid, while others believe they are detrimental to health.

Isoflavones are classified as phytoestrogens, named for the hormone estrogen. This means that they can have very mild estrogenic (estrogen enhancing) effects under some conditions and anti-estrogenic effects under others, as they block the body's hormonally active compounds. Because of this, soy isoflavones have been and continue to be studied to determine their relationship to conditions and diseases of particular concern to women.

There is not yet conclusive evidence about isoflavones, and they may in fact both help and hurt us, depending on how much we consume. What we do know is that isoflavones, like most natural nutrients, don't do anything bad to you if you don't eat too much of them.

In some Asian countries, people are estimated to consume 10 to 30 milligrams of isoflavones by eating tofu and miso every single day and suffer no consequences. In the United States, on the other hand, some people eat as much as 80 to 100 milligrams per day via soy shakes, soy energy bars, soy cereal, and a ton of other processed, reconstituted soy foods. You don't have to be a scientist to guess that OD'ing on this junk isn't going to do your body any favors.

The most common, accessible type of natural soy is tofu, which is what you get when you coagulate soy milk and press the remaining curds. Sound gross? It's not. It tastes mild and nutty, with a texture like scrambled eggs. In fact, tofu is a great stand-in for scrambled eggs. It comes in a variety of types, so you can choose anything from very soft and crumbly silken tofu all the way through very firm varieties with a texture like hard cheese. Softer is better for soups, but you'll want firmer varieties in your stir-fries. I love marinating and grilling a slab of very firm tofu and putting it on a whole wheat roll with lettuce and tomato for a burger. Tofu has a tendency to absorb the flavor of whatever it's eaten with, so go wild with it—there's almost nothing it can't complement.

As I say, like any other food, soy by itself won't cure all that ails you or make you live longer. But even without any magic nutrients, if you eat soy in place of meat, you'll be taking in less fat and calories. That alone makes it a heart-healthy food.

33

Eating "Aminals" Isn't Nice

The Reverend Martin Luther King Jr. once said, "One day the absurdity of the almost universal human belief in the slavery of other animals will be palpable. We shall then have discovered our souls and become worthier of sharing this planet with them."

The longer I've been on this "plant-tastic" journey, the more I realize how inexcusable it is that we eat animals. It's terrifyingly pathetic, sad, and completely unnecessary.

Did you know humans eat more than sixty billion animals each year? Sixty (swallow) billion!

To give you an idea of how many that is, I want you to think about this: One million seconds is the equivalent of thirteen days. One billion seconds is the equivalent of thirty-three years. Or, if you want a visual, strung together from head to hoof and beak to feet, all the animals that humans slaughter and then consume every year would stretch from the earth to the moon and back two-and-a-half times!

This is absolute carnage in the name of satisfying our insatiable addiction to unhealthful food. It is a display of selfishness, arrogance, elitism, and ignorance beyond reproach. And the more you know, the worse it gets. Hundreds of books have been written about the torture that farm animals must live through, but I won't go into it in depth here.

But in a nutshell, animals raised on typical industrial-style or "factory" farms lead excruciatingly miserable lives—almost beyond belief. Their existence is controlled from conception to consumption; they are treated like commodities, not living creatures. Chickens raised for meat are bred to grow so fast and large that millions die of heart attacks at just weeks old; they experience chronic pain as their legs struggle to support their unwieldy bodies. Millions of animals, such as calves raised for veal, sows used for breeding, and hens used in egg production, are packed into cages and crates so tightly that they can barely move—their entire lives are spent in a pen that restricts them from even stretching a limb.

Farm animals are routinely mutilated without painkillers: Pigs have their tails cut off, as do some dairy cows; egg-laying hens have parts of their beaks cut off; turkeys have parts of their beaks and toes cut off; and male cattle and pigs are castrated. At slaughterhouses, the kill line moves quickly and animals (particularly chickens) often are not adequately stunned unconscious, such that they are boiled or dismembered while still aware.

This is just the tip of the iceberg when it comes to the extraordinary cruelty we display in slaughtering these sixty billion creatures a year. Ask yourself: When I eat an animal, am I not basically condoning this kind of torture? And the United States has no federal laws to protect these poor creatures.

At this moment, the only person who can help stop these animals from being tortured and eaten is you. You and your family, that is. My now six-year-old son, Kole, and four-year-old daughter, Sophie, are at that adorable age when they only see the beauty, wonder, and good in the world. They have zero prejudices, and haven't yet developed any of the biases we hold as adults. They are the ones who can teach us—if we'll just listen.

Kole and Sophie don't understand why people eat animals. They love every animal from the hippo to the horse to the pig and the cow. The biggest and most popular field trip they take at their school is the one to Crow's Nest Farm to see the animals. Their favorite books, too, are the ones with animals in them: *The Cat in the Hat*, *Peter Rabbit*, *Charlotte's Web*, *The Story of Noah's Ark*...and many more.

When we gently let Kole and Sophie know that people eat pigs and cows and chickens in the form of hot dogs, hamburgers, and nuggets, they became sad and confused. We were recently at a grocery store and when we passed the meat section, Kole commented, "All the meat looks gross and bloody and they cut off the heads and I don't want people to kill the 'aminals' because the 'aminals' are nice. I don't get why people eat lambs, and gooses, and cows, and pigs, and chickens, and tigers, and fish."

Don't eat "aminals." Align your diet with your values: Eat plants, and leave the killing behind.

34

Eat Plants. Lose Weight. Feel Great.

As much as the diet industry wants you to believe that there are all kinds of fancy secrets to losing weight, there really is only one: Burn more calories than you take in and the pounds will come off.

And if you are attempting to do that by eating less and exercising more, you're just chasing your tail. And therein lies the beauty of eating plants. It's a formula that makes sense for many, many reasons.

When you eat whole, plant-based foods, you are eating calorie-light foods that are wonderfully bulky from water and fiber as well as layered with vitamins, minerals, and phytochemicals. When the bulk of the fiber, water, and micronutrients hits your stomach, it signals your body's stretch receptors and the nutrient receptors that all is well in the world. When you eat meat and processed foods, however, you are eating calorie-rich foods that are empty of fiber, water, and micronutrients and don't signal your stomach's density and stretch receptors until it's too late and you've overindulged—and still leave you micronutrient deficient.

Still, despite this easy formula, one in three American adults and one in six children are obese. There are many factors behind America's supersizing, including an increased consumption of processed and restaurant foods, but the heart of the problem is that people are simply eating too many calories—especially calories from meat, dairy, and processed foods, affectionately known as C.R.A.P.—calorie rich and processed—a term coined by my friend Jeff Novick.

A 2009 study by Johns Hopkins University found that participants who ate the most meat consumed 700 more calories every day than those who ate the least. They were also 27 percent more likely to be overweight.

On the other side of the equation are the plant eaters. According to a review of 87 studies published in the April 2006 edition of *Nutrition Reviews*, while obesity rates among meat eaters have skyrocketed, they've remained at between 0 and 6 percent among plant eaters. On top of that, the study found that the body weight of male and female plant eaters was 3 to 30 percent lower on average than that of meat eaters.

The reason is clear: Meat and other animal-based foods are usually loaded with fat. That's what made meat so handy as an occasional snack for our hunter-gatherer ancestors. Fatty, calorific foods are great if you spend all day running away from saber-toothed tigers and don't know when you will eat next, but not so great if spend your days staring at a computer screen and chowing down in restaurants. It's a simple fact: More sedentary lifestyles require diets with less fat and more plants, which are nature's low-fat wonders.

Let's look at the amount of fat in foods with and without meat. How about a great bowl of Bad 2 the Bone Chili (page 175)? Throw in some lentils, kidney beans, a load of tomatoes and other veggies and bam! This bowl contains around 1 to 2 grams of fat. The main sources are the lentils and the kidney beans, which pack a minuscule 0.71 grams, totaling just 3 percent of your overall calorie intake.

Now let's look at that bowl if you add one serving size of ground beef. It contains 22 grams of fat—a full 71 percent of the calories in the meat! Just by adding meat, you have created a dish nearly four times fattier than the original. And what's a meat-eater's bowl of chili without a good layer of cheese on top? Throw on a half cup of shredded cheddar for another 18 grams of fat. There is more fat in cheese than there is in the leaner types of ground beef!

You get the point. Anyone who says he or she doesn't feel full without meat simply hasn't eaten enough potatoes, brown rice, squash, black-eyed peas, or steel-cut oats—the bulk and fiber in these and other such foods (missing in meat) make you feel fuller on fewer calories.

None of this means that it's impossible to get fat if you eat only plants. In fact, if you eat nothing but French fries, fast-food salads with oily dressing, and lots of refined carbs such as white bread, you may well get as obese as any meat eater. The point is that plants in their natural state are low in calories, low in fat, high in fiber, high in water, and high in micronutrients, and if you eat them intelligently, the only thing you'll have to worry about growing big is your ego when you see how slim and trim you are.

35

Be Done with Dumb Diets

The dieting world is full of magic bullets. The reality is they are all piggies wearing different-colored lipstick: low-carb, no carb, all carb, dark carb, net carb, blood type, caveman, Paleo, primal, cookie, warrior, monk, and a dictionary full of other made-up names to go with made-up claims.

What do these diets have in common? They don't tend to work. The reason is simple: Most fad diets are based on calorie restriction (aka starving yourself). They dress it up in a lot of colorful costumes, but it usually boils down to the same strategy: Eat fewer calories than your daily requirement, and you will lose weight.

This is more or less true—as long as you don't read the fine print stating that you will gain all your weight back when you start eating normally again. One of the most comprehensive analyses of dieting ever done found that almost everyone who followed leading fad diets eventually gained back whatever weight they had lost within six months (other studies have found the weight comes back within two years).

In fact, in some of the studies, being on a diet almost guaranteed that over time, a person would actually gain more weight than they had lost!

The real problem with fad diets (well, outside of the fact that they don't work) is that they aren't designed to be healthy. They are designed to make you lose weight. But you can't keep the weight off unless you are eating healthily.

See where this is going?

Like a good soldier you follow the diet for a while, but eventually you break rank and return to overeating. Dieticians call this process "restriction-binge" cycles, and they lead to yo-yo dieting, or losing weight and gaining it back again...and again and again. This kind of weight loss has been linked to a weakened immune system, cardiovascular disease, hypertension, and diabetes.

The worst types of diets, such as crash diets, are starvation marathons with a bit of liquid allowed to fool your body into thinking it isn't cannibalizing itself. Although you initially lose weight, in the long term you don't because your body responds to starving by slowing your metabolism while eating into your muscles. Even when you start eating normally again, your metabolism remains depressed, causing you to gain more weight from less food. On top of that, these diets deprive you of vitamins and minerals, dehydrate you, and even weaken your heart.

Doing one once probably won't hurt you, but doing it multiple times (essentially yo-yo dieting) has been linked to an increased risk of heart attacks. One of the original liquid diets, the "Last Chance Diet," allowed for just 300 calories a day and was linked to sixty deaths from heart disease. As for the "cleansing" properties that these diets claim—well, hooey. That's what you have a liver and kidneys for.

Fad diets that often limit or nix healthy foods are almost always based on gaga theories demonizing one specific nutrient in order to convince you that cutting it out of your diet is all you need to lose weight.

Take carbohydrates. Even if you ignore the fact that cutting out carbs and eating more fat and protein directly contradicts almost all the published health studies of the last half century, it is still completely bananas to believe that you can eat as much fat as you want as long as you limit your carb intake. It's like saying you can smoke as much as you want, just stay away from sugar; that way you won't get diabetes. But you probably will get lung cancer. The same goes for "no-fat" diets that let you eat as many empty carbs as you want as long as they say "fat-free."

The truth is that fat, protein, carbohydrates, and all other nutrients are necessary in your diet, just not in excess. Removing any of them may help you shed weight, but will also add new problems. For example, despite the fact that most people who follow low-carb (or low anything) diets can't stick with them in the long term, they do cause dieters to lose pounds...if they're desperate enough. But most of the "pound a day" claims of low-carb diets are caused by dehydration. If that's not your style, they can also induce *ketosis*, which is a biological state that also happens in diabetics when they don't get enough insulin.

The biggest scams are the diets that come with a miracle food, like cookies, or supplement shakes, vinegar, or even hormones from the urine of pregnant women—I wish I were making that one up. Usually the people promoting these diets are—surprise!—the same people trying to get you to buy their miracle products. I can't tell you how many women have told me that they are "professional dieters" and are looking for something, anything, that works and is sustainable.

What makes plant-based eating any different? For starters, it's about eating, not starving. People on plant-based diets can eat lots and lots of delicious, wonderful food, but because the food is high in fiber and water content and low in calories, you'll fill up before you fill out.

Next, plant-based eating doesn't deny your body any nutrients in the name of weight loss. As long as you eat a nice variety of plants, you will get ample amounts of carbs, proteins, fats, vitamins, minerals, micro-nutrients, and everything else your body needs, but you won't get them in the excessive quantities that cause weight gain. For the first time in your life you'll be getting healthy and beautiful from the inside out, the natural side effect of which will be sustainable and permanent weight loss.

Finally, once you switch to a plant-based diet, you won't have to battle cravings or worry about your weight yo-yoing. That's because it is low in calories and high in nutrients, so you won't want to eat anything else. You will have a happy and heavenly relationship with your food!

Conclusion
Bring on the Plants!

I've been following a plant-strong diet for more than twenty-six years and I'm 100 percent convinced that it's the healthiest and most satisfying way to eat. But I know that few topics can rile people up as much as diet and food. I hope these chapters will give you all the information you need to flip meat eaters to plant eaters (especially if that meat eater is you!).

Collectively, we live in a society that still cherishes its meat. It will take some time before people come around to the benefits of eating plant-strong. Be patient. It will happen. You are a pioneer, an early adopter of a lifestyle that is becoming more and more prevalent. As Winston Churchill said, "America always gets it right, but only after they've tried everything else."

Plant-strong is a concept whose time has come, and I want to thank you for being an agent of change in transforming your health and the health of this country. Healthy citizens are the greatest asset any country can have!

On an individual level, this is a journey about building health. It all begins with eating whole, plant-based foods. Don't make this more complicated than it has to be. Let's not count calories; let's not obsess over portion sizes; let's not worry whether we're eating two, three, four, or six times a day; let's not make this about willpower. Let's make this about plant power, my broccoli brothers and strawberry sisters! Let's just make this about eating simple, whole, plant-based foods.

I want you to push out the processed and animal-based foods by piling up your plate with plants. This way you'll have zero room for anything else. I want to challenge you to have a plant-strong meal so big it needs its own zip code. I want you to explore how much you can eat of these clean, low-calorie foods before your tummy receptors decisively let you know you've had enough to eat. I want you to start mainlining the fruits, veggies, and legumes like they are your drugs of choice because guess what: they are!

Let's stop the human suffering and step up and challenge the doctors who keep people locked in the circle of insanity with drugs, surgery, endless tests and procedures, and a bad diet.

Don't be afraid of change. Let the plant-strong lifestyle show you a world where anything is possible—a world without prescription drugs, lethargy, ill-health, chronic disease, and sickness. Where you go from here is a choice I leave with you. Take it. It's yours!

And now on to the best part: the food. Coming up are more than 140 amazing recipes that are the cherry on top of the moo-free sundae— all plant-sensational, with healthy fats and no added oils. I've found that even if I don't always win my plant-strong argument—every now and then someone is stubborn—all I have to do is feed them, and suddenly a grin breaks over their faces and they see the plant-strong light! Split Figs with Cashew Cream and Caramelized Onions (page 149)! Anne's Pumpkin Muffins (page 145)! Bad 2 the Bone Chili (page 175)! Hold on to Your Hat Steel-Cut Oats with Kale (page 178)! Raise-the-Barn Butternut Squash–Vegetable Lasagna (page 199)! Grape Tomato, Fresh Mint, and Watermelon Ball Salad (page 238)! Bittersweet Chocolate Truffles (page 264)!

Here's a fact I've found to be always true: It's hard to lose an argument when you're stuffing your opponent's face with the best food on earth!

PART II

THE RECIPES

People always ask me how I was able to get a bunch of burger-munching, ice cream–scarfing, milk-guzzling Texas firefighters to eat a healthy, whole-food, plant-strong diet.

The answer is twofold. First: I used all the arguments that you've now read in the first part of this book. When you really know your plant-strong stuff, you don't lose an argument because the facts are all on your side. Firefighters love to argue, so believe me, we talked about food and nutrition more than we talked about almost anything else!

However, some people don't respond to facts. So in those cases I resorted to the second part of my strategy (and this book): I fed them delicious burgers, scrumptious pizzas, amazing fajitas, filling "meat" loaves, and extraordinary desserts—all of which were plant-strong. The guys didn't miss their old foods because these new versions taste sensational and make them feel great. And they couldn't argue anymore because their mouths were filled with seconds and thirds and, yes, fourths.

Think about it. If a firehouse full of good ol' boys in Austin, Texas, can do this, any house, and I mean *any* house, can do this. It's all about making and eating kickass food that everyone from housewives to firefighters, from kids to seniors will truly love!

My first book, *The Engine 2 Diet*, featured 125 recipes. Since it was published, I've been traveling all over the country pushing plants, and it seems as though everywhere I've gone E2ers have shown up with wonderful recipes. So when I decided to write this second book, I knew I wanted to include as many of them as possible.

To help me get it right, I recruited my amazing sister, Jane, to captain this section of the book. Jane is married to the great Brian Hart; together, they have three children, Bainon, Crile, and Zeb. Jane is also a registered nurse, a sex education teacher, a wellness instructor, and a plant-strong presenter and cook. Like me, Jane runs full throttle on that rocket fuel we call plants!

Together we put out the call to E2ers far and wide seeking even more great recipes. Holy Kale! The next thing we knew we were inundated with hundreds upon hundreds of suggestions. Eventually, Jane and I culled through the recipes submitted by enthusiastic friends, strangers, chefs, comedians, bloggers, vegans, raw foodies, vegetarians, librarians, nurses, academicians, doctors, family members, cookbook authors, and even firefighters!

It wasn't easy, but we finally narrowed the field down to 140 that best represented the Engine 2 criteria of being delicious, satisfying, simple, and, of course, plant-strong.

Then, over the past two years, Jane poured her heart, soul, and kitchen into testing each and every one of these recipes. I am 100 percent confident that you will not just like these dishes, you will love them! And in the true spirit of love, this food will love you right back, helping to guide your health into the stratosphere. Plant-strong all the way!

Note: All of the recipes in this book follow these guidelines:

- They are plant-strong! One hundred percent plant based, they contain no animal products or by-products.
- They contain no added extracted oils.
- They use little to no salt.
- They use minimally processed sweeteners (predominantly pure maple syrup or dates).
- They are simple and easy to prepare.

Breakfast

Rip's Big Bowl

Start Your Engines!

By Rip Esselstyn

I pledge allegiance to the plants
that come from Mother Earth,
and to the Big Bowl, for which it stands;
one breakfast, hearty, heaping, and whole,
with health benefits for all.

Prep time: 5 minutes • Serves 1

½ cup old-fashioned oats, raw and uncooked

½ cup Ezekiel 4:9 cereal (or equivalent; Kashi or Grape-Nuts brand)

½ cup bite-size shredded wheat

1 tablespoon ground flaxseed or chia seeds

1 small handful walnuts

1 small banana, sliced

⅓ cup blueberries (frozen or fresh)

A handful of raisins

Almond milk, as much as you prefer

The night before, place the oats and other cereals in a bowl and seal with a lid. In the morning, add the ground flaxseed or chia, walnuts, banana, blueberries, raisins, and almond milk. Grab a spoon and go—you are invincible!

Variations: Add cherries, strawberries, grapes, mango, pomegranate seedpods, fresh grapefruit wedges, or pecans for variety and fun!

Whole Banana Oatmeal

By Maria Torres

Our super-nanny, Maria Torres, made this for Kole and Sophie one morning. I was blown away by its simplicity and tastiness.

Prep time/cook time: 8 minutes • Serves 2 to 4

2 cups water

1 banana, peeled and smashed

1 cup old-fashioned rolled oats

While heating the water for the oatmeal, stir in the whole smashed banana. Once the banana is incorporated uniformly, add the oats. Cook until the oatmeal is the desired consistency and serve.

Variation: Try this with fresh strawberries, raspberries, or the fruit of your choice.

Savory Shiitake and Cheesy Oats

By Debbie Kastner

If you haven't checked out *Happy Healthy Long Life* online, you need to! It's written by Debbie Kastner, aka the Healthy Librarian, and she has the most incredible website, featuring up-to-date research delivered in layman's terms as well as plant-strong recipes like this powerhouse of a breakfast. A double dose of nitric oxide and vessel-boosting power from oats and spinach—it's crazy how much nutrition is in this breakfast bowl!

Prep time: 20 minutes • Serves 2 to 4

1 cup steel-cut oats
2 cups water or vegetable broth
1 cup unsweetened non-dairy milk
2 tablespoons nutritional yeast
2 dashes ground turmeric
1½ teaspoons Cajun or Southwest seasoning of choice
Freshly ground black pepper

Pinch or two chipotle powder (optional)
1 ounce julienned sun-dried tomatoes
5 dried shiitake mushrooms, broken into pieces (or other dried mushrooms you like)
2½ ounces fresh baby spinach per serving

In a medium pot, mix the oats, water (or broth), non-dairy milk, nutritional yeast, turmeric, seasoning, black pepper to taste, chipotle powder, if using, sun-dried tomatoes, and mushrooms. Watching carefully, bring to a boil, reduce the heat, and simmer for about 10 minutes. Cook until all of the water is absorbed, leaving the oats nice and creamy.

When the oats are done, microwave 1 serving of spinach briefly until soft but not mushy, about 30 seconds. Top each serving of oatmeal with a portion of the softened spinach, mix, and enjoy. Store the remaining oatmeal in the fridge—it is easy to reheat in the microwave or on the stove top.

Variation: Instead of sun-dried tomatoes, substitute 3 times the amount of dried shiitake mushrooms. Serve over a bed of cooked kale with Jane's Dancing Dressing (page 214).

The Machu Picchu

By Rip and Jane Esselstyn

Quinoa is a high-protein, nutty-flavored ancient Incan grain. Prepare your quinoa the night before to save time in the morning. It can even be made in a rice cooker! Be sure to rinse it well to remove the natural *sopanios*, which can taste bitter or soapy. Other than that—

Any berries will do.

Any color quinoa will do.

Any nut butter—a little dab—will do.

Prep time: 5 minutes • Serves 1

¾ cup quinoa (red, white, or black), cooked

1 handful fresh blueberries, other berries, or fruit of choice

1 teaspoon peanut butter, almond butter, or nut butter of choice

Prepare the quinoa as directed on the package. The ratio is usually 1 cup quinoa to 2 cups water. Place the warm (or cold) cooked quinoa in a breakfast bowl and add the berries on top. Stir in the nut butter of choice.

Tip: If you are a big breakfast eater, use more quinoa and add a sliced banana to the mix.

Spicy Southern Grits

*By John Mercer, head prepared-foods chef at the
Park Lane, Texas, Whole Foods Market store*

My first experience with grits was at a summer camp when I was in the seventh grade. I took one spoonful of the warm, gelatinous mixture and thought I was going to lose it. I tried them again in college with a very similar reaction. Now that I have a much more sophisticated and discerning palate, I appreciate and devour these spicy grits!

Prep time: 20 minutes • Serves 4

1 small yellow onion, diced

1 tablespoon garlic, minced

¼ cup green chilies, diced

1 chipotle pepper, chopped

2 cups vegetable stock

½ cup yellow grits

3 tablespoons nutritional yeast

Juice of ½ lime

½ teaspoon salt (optional)

1 teaspoon freshly ground black pepper (optional)

In a medium pot over high heat, sauté the onions, garlic, green chilies, and chipotle pepper with 2 tablespoons of the stock for 5 to 7 minutes. Add the remaining stock and bring to a boil. Whisk in the grits and cook over low heat for 5 to 7 minutes, whisking occasionally until thick and well absorbed. Stir in nutritional yeast and lime.

Taste and adjust the seasoning to your liking, add the salt, if using, and serve.

Tip: This is fantastic for dinner served with Grilled Thai Kale Salad (page 239) on top!

The Bouldin Creek Spicy Scrambler

By Leslie and the Bouldin Creek Café staff

The Bouldin Creek Café is an ultra-cool, newly renovated, totally badass, plant-based restaurant in South Austin. This scrambled tofu is one of their signature dishes, and a favorite when my wife, Jill, and I decide to go out for plant-strong fare. We always ask them to top our salads with it. The owner, Leslie, was kind enough to share her most beloved secret recipe.

Press time: 30 minutes • Prep time/cook time: 10 minutes (plus 30 minutes press time for tofu) • Serves 3 to 4

TOFU

> One 12-ounce block firm tofu
> 1 to 2 teaspoons low-sodium tamari sauce or Bragg Liquid Aminos

SPICY MIX

> ½ jalapeño pepper, finely chopped
> ½ serrano pepper, finely chopped
> 1 garlic clove, minced
> ½ cup chopped fresh cilantro

DRY MIX

> 1 teaspoon curry powder
> ¼ teaspoon salt (optional)
> ¼ teaspoon ground turmeric
> ½ teaspoon freshly ground black pepper
> 1 cup nutritional yeast

Wrap the block of tofu in a dish towel and place it in a colander over a bowl. Press it for at least 30 minutes using something heavy, like a brick or carton of non-dairy milk. (This is an important step or your tofu will come out gummy!)

In a small bowl, create the spicy mix. Combine the jalapeño and serrano peppers, garlic, and cilantro. Combine the curry powder, salt, turmeric, black pepper, and nutritional yeast in a heated nonstick pan. Crumble the tofu with your hands into jagged, bite-size pieces—it will look like scrambled eggs! Add a splash of tamari or Bragg Liquid Aminos and stir to incorporate. Add the tofu to the dry mix and stir until uniformly coated—it may look like there is too much dry mix—just keep stirring it around and it will all cling to the tofu eventually. Add the spicy mix and sauté until the peppers and tofu are heated through.

Serve warm on its own, or use as a filling for breakfast tacos, burritos, or enchiladas. Also try it in a shepherd's pie, or paired with greens like kale or Swiss chard!

Real Flapjacks

By Jane Esselstyn

Real flapjacks come from the United Kingdom and they are simple as can be. They are not flour-based or pan-cooked like American pancakes; they are more like sweet oat squares. According to my sister, Jane, who is obsessed with Scotland, "This is a real Scottish breakfast for ye wee lads and lassies. Pack a stash in your sporran and they'll keep yer stride long all day o'er the highlands, and to the bonnie, bonnie banks o' Loch Lomond."

Prep time: 5 minutes • Cooking time: 25 minutes • Cooling time: 10 minutes • Makes 12 oat squares

⅔ cup raw cashews or walnuts

2 tablespoons water

⅓ cup pure maple syrup

1⅓ cups old-fashioned rolled oats

½ teaspoon vanilla extract

¼ teaspoon ground cinnamon

⅓ cup total: dried cranberries, raisins, dried cherries, pistachios, almonds, or pecans (optional)

Preheat the oven to 350°F. Line a shallow 9 x 11-inch pan with parchment paper.

Place the nuts in a food processor with the water and grind, scraping the sides down if needed, until it forms a big clump.

Add the maple syrup, vanilla, and cinnamon and process until well combined. Hand mix or gently pulse the oats into the mix. Add the optional ingredients, if using, at this stage. Press the oat mixture into the lined pan until flat and about ¼ inch thick. Bake for 25 minutes, or until golden around the edges.

Remove from the oven and, while still warm, score the surface to mark 12 or 16 pieces. Set aside to cool. When cooled completely, about 20 minutes, cut with a sharp knife. Serve crispy, crunchy, and cool.

Tips: Use this mixture as a crumble topping over Apple-Cardamom Flap-jack Crumble (page 257). Also, use as a piecrust by pressing into a pie plate and baking as above.

Dinosaur Gingerbread-Buckwheat Pancakes

Inspired by A-K @ Swell Vegan Blog

The Esselstyn family loves making pancakes on the weekends. The only animals we eat in our house are the bunnies or dinosaurs that Jill makes for the kids out of pancake batter. And I've always prided myself on turning pancakes the size of manhole covers with the flip of a wrist. Kole gets so excited wanting to flip pancakes the way Daddy does that we got him a pint-size frying pan so he can get in on the action while Sophie cheers. The lucky recipient of any pancakes that land on the floor is our eleven-year-old Queensland Heeler, Tug.

Prep time/cook time: 10 minutes • Makes 4 to 5 medium pancakes

¼ cup buckwheat flour

½ cup gluten-free flour mix

1 tablespoon ground flaxseed

½ tablespoon baking powder

¾ teaspoon ground ginger

½ teaspoon ground cinnamon

¼ teaspoon ground cardamom

⅛ teaspoon ground nutmeg

⅛ teaspoon ground cloves

¼ teaspoon salt

⅓ cup unsweetened non-dairy milk

⅓ cup water

3 tablespoons pure maple syrup

1 teaspoon vanilla extract

In a medium bowl, whisk together the flours, flaxseed, baking powder, and spices. Make a well in the center of the mix.

In a small bowl, whisk together the milk, water, maple syrup, and vanilla and pour into the dry ingredients' well. Mix together with a spoon or silicone spatula. Let the mixture rest 5 to 10 minutes to allow the liquids to absorb into the flour; the mixture will probably be thicker and goopier than traditional pancake batter.

Heat a skillet over medium heat, and add ¼ to ⅓ cup of the batter per pancake, spreading them out into a circle. Cook 3 to 4 minutes until the edges firm up and the tops begin to dry out, then flip over and cook on the opposite side for 1 to 2 minutes more. Serve immediately, or keep warm on a plate in the oven.

Berry Berry Good Sauce

Inspired by Chef Marco and Karime

Jane and I ran into this sauce in the Texas hill country during an Engine 2 retreat, and we find it replaces maple syrup atop our breakfast favorites. It is delicious on Dinosaur Gingerbread-Buckwheat Pancakes (page 143), Cranberry-Polenta French Toast (page 147), or even on Rip's Big Bowl (page 138). Use any kind of berries that you prefer: raspberry, blueberry, blackberry, or strawberry!

Prep time: 10 minutes • Makes 2 cups

> 1½ cups berries (your choice: raspberry, blueberry, blackberry, or strawberry)
> ½ cup orange juice (makes it more sour) *or* apple juice (makes it more sweet)

Over high heat, in a medium saucepan boil your choice of berries and juice for 5 minutes. It will become more syrup-like as it cooks. Remove the sauce from the heat and pour it into a blender or food processor. Blend until the sauce is syrup-like with a bit of fruit still visible, then serve and enjoy.

Tip: If you choose strawberries for your sauce, boil them for only 3 to 4 minutes because the berries lose their redness if they cook too long.

Zeb's Waffles

By Zeb Esselstyn

These are the most dense and hearty waffles I've ever had in my life. My mom and my brother, Zeb, have had a running contest for the last year to see who could make the best waffle. The inspiration was to turn the Rip's Big Bowl cereal concoction (see page 138) into a waffle. Zeb's recipe wins!

Prep time: 10 minutes • Cook time: 5 minutes • Makes 4 square waffles

> 2½ cups old-fashioned rolled oats
> ¾ cup finely chopped walnuts
> ¼ cup flaxseed meal
> Zest of ½ orange
>
> ½ to ¾ teaspoon ground cinnamon
> 1 medium banana, smashed
> 1 to 1½ cups almond milk

Preheat a waffle iron.

In a bowl, combine the oats, walnuts, flaxseed meal, orange zest, and cinnamon. Place two-thirds of the mixture into a food processor or high-speed blender. Blend until the mixture has a flour-like texture. Return to the bowl with the remaining one-third of the dry ingredients; this step ensures that the waffles have a chunky texture. If you prefer a smoother, uniform texture to your waffles, blend all of the dry ingredients initially.

Add the smashed banana and almond milk to the dry ingredients in the bowl. Mix thoroughly with a fork; the batter will be fairly thick. If you prefer a thinner batter, add more almond milk.

Portion the batter thickly onto a preheated waffle iron and spread it out to all corners. Close the lid, and cook the waffle according to the manufacturer's directions for your waffle iron. When done, remove the waffle from the iron—some waffles require the assistance of a chopstick to encourage release from the waffle iron. Top with the fruit of choice and/or syrup and serve.

Tip: These rule. Make the whole batch over the weekend, freeze any extras, and microwave one for a midweek breakfast on the go.

Anne's Pumpkin Muffins

By Anne Stevenson

Anne Stevenson is an artist, graphic designer, mother of three, IronMan triathlete, and plant-strong baking ninja as well! On top of all that, she is the woman who posed with me in the exercise section of my book *The Engine 2 Diet*. Whenever she brings these muffins to our monthly potluck, they are gone lickety-split.

Prep time: 10 minutes • Makes 12 muffins

One 14-ounce can pure pumpkin puree (no sugar added)

2 ripe bananas, mashed

1 cup unsweetened applesauce

2 to 3 dashes pumpkin pie spice

1 teaspoon vanilla extract

3 cups oat flour

1 teaspoon baking soda

1 teaspoon baking powder

½ teaspoon sea salt (optional)

Preheat the oven to 350°F. Set out a silicone muffin tray or nonstick 12-well muffin pan.

In a large bowl, stir together the pumpkin, bananas, applesauce, pumpkin pie spice, and vanilla. In a separate bowl, combine the oat flour, baking soda, baking powder, and salt.

Combine the wet and dry ingredients. Spoon the batter into the muffin pan. Bake for 33 minutes. Set aside to cool for a few minutes; they should pop out of the muffin pan very easily.

Tip from Anne: These muffins are best served warm! The recipe can be modified depending on the time of year or the ingredients you have on hand. Sometimes I push a blackberry into each muffin before I bake them, or add chocolate chips—for dessert muffins!

A-2-Z Muffins

By Katherine Lawrence

These muffins are the creation of Katherine Lawrence with The Cancer Project in Dallas, Texas. She created them at the behest of her family to make a healthy muffin that no one could resist. These are low fat, guilt-free, tasty, and easy to eat on the go.

Prep time: 15 minutes • Cook time: 45 minutes • Makes 12 muffins

¼ cup ground flaxseed
⅓ cup hot water
½ cup applesauce
⅓ cup pure maple syrup
1 teaspoon vanilla extract
1 cup grated carrot
1 cup grated zucchini

1 red apple, grated
1¾ cups whole wheat pastry flour
2 teaspoons baking powder
1 teaspoon ground cinnamon
½ teaspoon salt (optional)
½ cup chopped walnuts (optional)

Preheat the oven to 350°F. Set out a silicone muffin tray or nonstick 12-well muffin pan.

Add the ground flaxseed and hot water to a cup and stir together with a fork. Allow to sit for 5 minutes until the mixture thickens to an egg-like consistency. In a large bowl, mix together the applesauce, maple syrup, and vanilla. Stir in the grated carrot, zucchini, and apple.

In a separate bowl, mix together the flour, baking powder, cinnamon, and salt. Stir the flaxseed mixture into the wet mixture, then add the dry mixture to the wet mixture and stir until well incorporated.

Spoon the batter into the muffin tray or pan and top with the chopped walnuts, if using. Bake for 40 to 45 minutes until the muffins are baked through; the muffins should be moist and chewy.

Note: In some ovens these muffins bake better at 425°F for 25 minutes.

Cranberry-Polenta French Toast

By Ben Baker

This polenta French toast is the mastermind of Ben Baker of the Travassa Spa and Resort, located in the Texas hill country (where we have held several of our Engine 2 retreats). Ben came up with this wonderful recipe for our gluten-free, plant-strong participants. It serves its purpose as good ol'-fashioned comfort food.

Prep time: 10 minutes • Cooling time: as little as 30 minutes to as long as overnight • Cook time: 5 minutes • Serves 6 to 12

- 3 cups water
- ¼ teaspoon ground cinnamon
- 2 tablespoons pure maple syrup
- 1 cup polenta
- 1 cup dried cranberries (about 5 ounces)

Add the 3 cups of water to a small pot. Whisk in the cinnamon and maple syrup very well, breaking up any clumps. Bring the mixture to a low boil.

Following the package instructions and using the suggested polenta-to-water ratio (some varieties are of a coarser grind and will absorb more water), whisk the water and slowly pour in the polenta. Cook, stirring rapidly, to keep the polenta from forming lumps. When the polenta has thickened like a nice porridge, stir in the cranberries.

Pour the mixture onto a baking sheet with a rim at least 1 inch high. Spread out the mixture to a thickness of less than ½ inch, making it as smooth as possible. Place a piece of parchment paper on the top of the smooth surface, and press the polenta flat. Allow the polenta to cool down, then refrigerate.

Once the polenta has set, you can unmold it onto a flat, clean surface. Cut it into even squares, and then cut the squares into triangles. Over medium-high heat, cook the triangles on each side in a nonstick pan until they turn golden brown. Serve plain, or with pure maple syrup, berries, or try Ben's magic trick below.

Ben's Baker Tip: Top with Cabernet Cranberries. In a small pot over medium heat, combine 2 cups of Cabernet wine with 1½ cups dried cranberries. Cook, letting the mixture slowly reduce, and until the cranberries have absorbed all of the wine. The pectin that still resides in the cranberries will cause the mixture to thicken. Drizzle the sauce over your Polenta French Toast—you are in for a real treat!

Sides and Appetizers

Split Figs with Cashew Cream and Caramelized Onions

By Anne Bingham

Near our family farm in upstate New York, tucked between the Berkshire and Catskill mountains, is a little natural-food grocery called Guido's. Shopping there one perfect summer day, my sister-in-law Anne came across a sample table offering several dishes with amazing blends of flavors. After taste-testing nearly all of their samples, she headed home to re-create this plant-strong version!

Prep time: 15 minutes (plus 30 minutes for soaking cashews) • Serves 6 to 8

    ½ cup raw cashews
    1 red onion, sliced
    ¼ teaspoon salt or low-sodium tamari sauce
    ¼ cup water, as needed
    6 to 8 fresh figs

Soak the cashews in a bowl of water for 30 minutes.

Place a sauté pan over high heat until a drop of water beads across the preheated surface. Add the red onion slices and cook until browned and caramelized. Set aside.

To make the cashew cream: Combine the drained cashews, salt or tamari, and water in a food processor and blend until creamy.

Without cutting all the way through, split figs into quarters—length- and width-wise—then open them out flat like stars. Spoon a dab of the cashew cream in the center of each split fig. Cover with the caramelized red onions. Serve cold or at room temperature with plenty of napkins.

Kitty's First Course

Adapted from a Crile family recipe

Kitty was a full-time cook for my great-grandparents' household nearly one hundred years ago. Whatever she cooked, the family loved. Her "first course" was heavenly, and perhaps helped send a few people in that direction since it included white bread, egg whites, mayonnaise, hollandaise sauce, grated egg yolk, and caviar. Gulp! Here is our E2, plant-strong, equally heavenly, and healthier version.

Prep time: 15 minutes • Serves 6

6 slices whole-grain bread, each cut into a 3½-inch diameter circle

6 artichoke bottoms—not hearts! (available canned)

2 cups steamed greens: kale, beet greens, Swiss chard, spinach— your choice

6 thick tomato slices, cut roughly the diameter of the toast rounds

½ cup OMG Walnut Sauce (page 216)

Kelp flakes, or fresh cilantro leaves, for garnish

Using the circular rim of a cup or cutter, cut the bread into 6 circles. Toast the bread circles.

On top of each round of toast, place an artichoke bottom. On top of each artichoke bottom, place ¼ cup of steamed greens. On top of the greens, add a tomato slice.

Prepare the walnut sauce and add water until the sauce has the consistency of a dressing. Spoon the sauce over the top of each "tower." Sprinkle with kelp flakes or cilantro. Enjoy!

ACE's Original Hummus-Collard Wraps

By Ann Esselstyn

These are bold, bright, fresh, and alive, just like my mom, Ann Crile Esselstyn (aka ACE), who created them.

Prep time: 15 minutes • Serves 4 to 6

4 collard greens (tips of stems removed so they are round)

½ cup hummus (see variation Plain Jane Hummus, page 221)

3 to 4 scallions, chopped

1 red bell pepper, julienned

1 small cucumber, peeled, seeded, and sliced lengthwise into ½-inch strips

4 to 6 leaves fresh basil, chopped

⅓ cup fresh cilantro, chopped

Zest and juice of 1 lemon

Lightly steam the collard leaves in a shallow pan of water for 10 seconds per side. Flatten out the steamed greens on a clean dish towel and dry both sides. Place one collard on a cutting board and coat the center spine thickly with the hummus.

Along the center strip of hummus, add the scallions, bell pepper, and cucumber strips atop the hummus. Add the basil, cilantro, lemon zest, and plenty of lemon juice. Roll up each collard green so each looks like a thick green cigar, then slice into ½-inch sections and serve.

Tip: Also try these using bok choy strips and asparagus!

Asparagus and Cream of Cashew Collard Wraps

By Jane Esselstyn

Asparagus and cashew cream are Jane's twist on my mom's Original Hummus-Collard Wraps. One rainy day while Jane was offering demos at a farmers' market, a young man tasted a collard wrap sample and shouted, "No way! What is this? I need this recipe!" Ask and ye shall receive.

Prep time: 15 minutes (plus 30 minutes for soaking the cashews) • Serves 4 to 6

½ cup raw cashews, soaked
¼ teaspoon salt
¼ cup water, or as needed
½ red onion, sliced
6 asparagus spears, steamed
4 collard greens, tips of stems removed so they are round

1 small cucumber, peeled, seeded, and sliced lengthwise
1 red bell pepper, julienned
3 to 4 scallions, chopped
4 to 6 leaves fresh basil, chopped
⅓ cup chopped fresh cilantro
Zest and juice of 1 lemon

In a food processor make cashew cream. Combine the soaked cashews, salt, and water and process until the texture is similar to hummus. Place a pan over high heat until a drop of water beads across the preheated surface. Add the red onion slices until browned and caramelized. Set aside.

In a shallow pan of water, lightly steam the asparagus. Set aside.

In the same pan of hot water, lightly steam the collard greens, about 10 seconds per side. Flatten out steamed greens on a clean dish towel and dry both sides.

Place one green on the cutting board at a time and coat the center spine thickly with cashew cream. Add a few cooked asparagus spears, cucumbers, bell peppers, and scallions atop the cashew cream. Sprinkle with the chopped basil and cilantro, lemon zest, and plenty of lemon juice. Roll collard green up so it looks like a thick green cigar. Repeat for the rest of the collard greens, then slice each into ½-inch sections and serve.

Spicy Italian Eat Balls

By Jane Esselstyn

Add these to pasta night and have an absolute ball! You can also serve them with toothpicks as hors d'oeuvres and watch them disappear. If you like things less spicy, use less Italian seasoning.

Prep time: 10 minutes • Cook time: 30 minutes • Makes about 20 to 40, depending on the size of the balls

¾ cup vegetable broth

1 tablespoon low-sodium tamari sauce

1 fresh garlic clove, minced

1 cup wheat gluten

1 to 2 tablespoons Italian seasoning

1 teaspoon dried oregano

¼ teaspoon garlic salt (optional)

1 teaspoon onion powder

2 tablespoons nutritional yeast

1 cup Fast and Fresh Marinara Sauce (page 227)

Preheat the oven to 375°F. Line a roasting pan with a layer of parchment paper.

In a small bowl, whisk together the broth, tamari, and garlic. In a separate bowl, mix together the wheat gluten, Italian seasoning, oregano, garlic salt, if using, onion powder, and nutritional yeast.

Combine the wet and dry ingredients. Hand mix and/or knead ingredients until there is an elastic texture to the dough. Using your hands, roll the dough into balls the size of grapes, walnuts, or golf balls. Place the balls onto the lined pan and baste with 1 cup of the marinara sauce. Bake for 20 minutes.

Remove from the oven, and, using a fork, rotate and roll the balls around, basting the tops and sides with the marinara in the pan. Bake for 10 minutes more. Remove from oven and serve warm over pasta with the remaining sauce.

Soulful BBQ Black-eyed Peas

Adapted from Bryant Terry's Vegan Soul Kitchen

After a long chat with my dad and mom, the producers of the documentary *Forks Over Knives* decided that as part of the movie they needed to film the story of a type 2 diabetic following a plant-strong diet. The woman they found was San'Dera Nation, a 300-pound, type 2 diabetic single mother of five who had little to lose by deciding to accept the challenge.

So, as cameras rolled, San'Dera started the plant-perfect way on Mother's Day of 2009. It was tough at first, but her near-immediate results—plummeting weight and blood sugar levels—made her stick with the plant-based approach. Now, more than a year later, San'Dera is 100 pounds lighter, no longer diabetic, and off her medications, and she feels great.

There are still challenges, however. Some of her African-American friends told her, "You're eating white food." Her response was, "I am eating healthy food. Not white people food or black people food, healthy food. I want to be around to play with my grans."

Here is a plant-soulful healthy favorite adapted from Bryant Terry and inspired by San'Dera's courage and resolve to rise above the fray.

Prep time: 10 minutes • Cook time: 15 minutes • Serves 8

1 medium onion, diced

2 garlic cloves, minced

1 green bell pepper, diced

Two 15-ounce cans black-eyed peas, drained and rinsed

10 ounces tempeh, chopped into small cubes (optional)

One 16-ounce jar barbecue sauce, your favorite

Preheat the oven to 350°F. In a cast-iron skillet, or other oven-safe cookware, cook the onion, garlic, and bell pepper over high heat until soft.

Decrease the heat to medium, add the black-eyed peas and tempeh, if using, and stir to combine. Add the barbecue sauce and stir until ingredients are uniformly coated with the sauce.

Place the pan into the oven and bake for 15 minutes, or until heated through. Serve warm on its own, over rice, or atop steamed greens.

Green Superheroes with Walnut Sauce or Balsamic Glaze

By Rip and Jane Esselstyn

The Justice League, from the comic book world, includes a lineup of superheroes. Our Justice League from the plant world includes kale, collards, bok choy, napa cabbage, spinach, mustard greens, beet greens, Swiss chard, broccoli, Brussels sprouts, and any other green leafy vegetable! This is a staple for any meal, even breakfast. Become a stripper of green leafy vegetables (see below for the proper Engine 2 technique) and watch your energy rise as your weight falls!

Prep time: 5 minutes • Cook time: 5 minutes • Serves 4 to 5

> 1 to 2 bunches kale, or greens of choice (about 4 cups)
> 1 cup OMG Walnut Sauce (page 216) or a balsamic glaze

Strip spines off of kale leaves and rinse them well.

Place the kale leaves in a pot with an inch or two of water and cook/steam until tender, about 3 to 5 minutes.

In a food processor, make the walnut sauce.

Serve the kale warm or cold topped with the OMG Walnut Sauce or a balsamic glaze such as Isola Classic Cream of Balsamic (see below).

Tip 1: The walnut sauce can be drizzled, poured, or spread on the greens, depending on how much water is added.

Tip 2: The balsamic glaze refers to Isola Classic Cream of Balsamic, or a similar product; it's a deceptive name, as there is no cream in it!

Note: To remove those thick spines magically from collard greens and kale: Hold the spine firmly in your dominant hand. Loosely hold the lower part of the spine just below the leafy greens in the other hand. (With some kale, you may need to tear back the lower leaves to expose some of the stem.) Holding firmly with the dominant hand, slide your other hand up the spine. You are left with all the greens in your opposite hand and the bare stem in dominant hand.

No-Moo-Here Mashed Potatoes

By Ann Esselstyn

My mom has taken one of the most wonderfully simple comfort-food side dishes and made it plant-a-licious without using butter or milk. No moo here!

Prep time: 40 minutes • Serves 6 to 8

> 6 medium Yukon Gold potatoes (for maximum nutrients, do not peel!)
> 1 to 2 cups non-dairy milk
> 2 to 4 tablespoons nutritional yeast, or as needed
>
> Salt
> Freshly ground black pepper
> 1 teaspoon garlic powder or garlic granules

Cut the unpeeled potatoes into small chunks, put into a large pot, and cover with water. Boil until tender, about 10 minutes. Drain the potatoes and transfer to a bowl.

Using an electric beater, beat the potatoes while adding non-dairy milk until you reach the desired smooth consistency; the potatoes may need more liquid than you might expect. Mix in nutritional yeast, salt and pepper to taste, and garlic powder. Serve warm.

Tip: For variety: Cook some Swiss chard, kale, or leafy green of choice in an inch of water until soft. Drain and stir into the potatoes. Nice GREEN potatoes! Or sprinkle in chopped scallions.

Better-milk Biscuits

By Jane Esselstyn

There is no *butter*-milk, just *better*-milk, in these biscuits: oat, almond, soy, or hazelnut milk! They are much better than the cow-based thing.

Prep time: 10 minutes • Cook time: 11 minutes • Makes 8 biscuits

2 cups white whole wheat flour, plus ½ cup for dusting the board

¼ teaspoon baking soda

1 tablespoon baking powder

½ teaspoon salt

⅔ cup raw, unsalted cashews or walnuts

2 tablespoons water

1 cup oat milk (or almond, soy, or hazelnut milk)

Preheat the oven to 400°F. Line a baking sheet with parchment paper, or use an aerated pan.

Combine the 2 cups flour, baking soda, baking powder, and salt in a bowl. In a food processor, blend the cashews and water until they form a dry clump of cashew butter. Remove the cashew butter from the food processor (no need to clean it yet!), and place in a small bowl.

Add the dry ingredients to the food processor. Crumble the cashew butter uniformly on top of the dry ingredients. Pulse the food processor a few times until the mixture has a mealy consistency; start with about 8 quick pulses. Add the oat milk and mix until just combined, no more.

Turn the dough out onto a floured board. Gently pat the dough out with your hands—not a rolling pin—until it's a thickness of about ½ inch. Gently and lightly fold the dough about 5 times over itself. Gently, press down on the dough until it is 1 inch thick. Using a round cutter, about 2 to 2½ inches in diameter—a drinking glass will also do—cut the dough into rounds. Knead scraps together to make more rounds and use up all the dough. If you prefer soft sides on your biscuits, place the biscuits on a cookie sheet touching each other; if you prefer crusty sides, place them about 1 inch apart.

Bake for 11 minutes. Serve warm plain, with fruit spreads, or with any soup from the soup section (page 245).

Tip: The key to really good biscuits is not in the ingredients, but in handling the dough as little as possible. Try baking these on an aerated cookie sheet for biscuits that are crispy on both the top and bottom. Try using other flours, as well. Or smother these with Mommy's Mushroom Gravy (page 218).

Lime-Ginger Tofu Cubes

Adapted from Clean Start *by Terry Walters*

The last Thursday of every month, Jill and I host a plant-strong potluck to introduce people to the E2 lifestyle as well as to show support for the growing E2 community in Austin, Texas. I recommend you do something similar. The delicious dishes people bring will blow you away and keep people coming back time and time again.

Prep time: 10 minutes • Serves 4

>   One 12-ounce package firm or extra-firm tofu (not silken!)
>   3 tablespoons fresh lime juice
>   2 tablespoons low-sodium tamari sauce
>   2 tablespoons pure maple syrup
>   1 tablespoon, plus 1 teaspoon peeled and minced fresh ginger

Slice the tofu into 1½-inch by ½-inch cubes. In a small bowl, combine the lime juice, tamari, and maple syrup.

In a nonstick pan over medium heat, cook the ginger for about 2 minutes until it browns slightly. Add the tofu cubes and tamari-lime-maple syrup mixture to the pan. Increase the heat to medium-high and cook for 4 to 5 minutes, stirring the cubes the entire time. Serve warm or cold.

Armadillo Sweet Potatoes

By Jane Esselstyn

Sweet potatoes prepared this way look remarkably like Texas armadillos. Serve a burnt-orange armada of armadillos to the kids (or adults) and watch them get gobbled up!

Prep time: 5 minutes • Cook time: 45 minutes • Serves 1 to 3, depending on the size of the sweet potato

> 1 sweet potato
> 1 fresh garlic clove, sliced as thinly as possible (optional)
> Crushed fresh herbs of your choice: oregano, rosemary, thyme, etc.

Preheat the oven to 400°F.

Slice the sweet potato in deep, horizontal, parallel slices—the pattern will resemble an armadillo's armor. Do not let the knife cut all the way to the base of the potato, just three-quarters of the way down. If you wish, squeeze in a sliver of garlic and the herbs of your choice in between the slices.

Cover with aluminum foil. Bake for 45 minutes. Serve on its own, or with Cilantro-Lime Pesto (page 230) or OMG Walnut Sauce (page 216) drizzled within the chinks of the Armadillo armor.

Fire Brigade Stuffing

By Brian Hart

My brother-in-law, Brian, makes this stuffing, which will make your palate swoon and your tummy sing. Here's a fun twist to make your guests swoon as well: Cook, then serve this inside a pumpkin. Seriously! Find a cooking pumpkin that will fit inside your oven, clean out the insides, stuff the open space with stuffing, place the lid back on, and cook as described below.

Prep time: 20 minutes • Cook time: 60 minutes • Serves 16 to 20

> 15 pieces of bread: 5 rye, 5 pumpernickel, and 5 whole wheat, cut into small cubes
> 1 large onion, diced
> 3 cups chopped celery
> 2 cups slivered carrots
> Two 16-ounce packages mushrooms, sliced
> 4 to 6 cups vegetable broth
> 1 Granny Smith apple, diced
> 1 red apple, diced
> 1 cup dried cranberries (about 5 ounces)
> 7 ounces almonds, slivered
> 2 to 3 tablespoons dried sage
> 2 teaspoons dried thyme
> 1 tablespoon dried oregano
> ½ teaspoon salt (optional)
> 1 teaspoon garlic powder
> ½ teaspoon freshly ground black pepper
> ½ to 1 cup tawny port

Preheat the oven to 350°F.

Place the cubed bread on a baking sheet and bake for about 15 minutes to dry it out, checking frequently to make sure it is not browning too much. Set aside.

In a sauté pan over medium-high heat, sauté the onion, celery, carrots, and mushrooms in ½ cup of the vegetable broth until softened. In a large bowl, combine the toasted bread cubes, cooked vegetables, apples, cranberries, almonds, sage, thyme, oregano, salt, if using, garlic powder, and pepper. Add broth and port to bowl as needed. Blend and toss until uniformly mixed and soggy.

Transfer the moist stuffing to lasagna pan (or a carved-out pumpkin). Cover with aluminum foil (or the pumpkin lid). Bake for 45 minutes to 1 hour. Serve warm with Down Under Cranberry Salsa (page 243).

Brussels Sprouts with Game

By Adrienne and Eric Hart

Brussels sprouts have little "game." Their naturally bitter flavor turns many people off from these leafy green, nutrient-power-packed balls of goodness. This dish has big-time game and will help the most die-hard Brussels sprouts haters get onboard the bandwagon. Game on!

Prep time: 10 minutes • Cook time: 20 minutes • Serves 4 to 6

   2½ to 3 cups Brussels sprouts, stemmed and halved lengthwise
   ⅓ cup pure maple syrup
   Freshly ground black pepper

Preheat the oven to 350°F. Line a baking dish with parchment paper.

Toss all three ingredients in a bowl until Brussels sprouts are well coated. Spread the Brussels sprouts out evenly in the lined baking dish. For softer Brussels sprouts, cover with aluminum foil and bake for 20 minutes. For firmer Brussels sprouts, bake, uncovered, for 25 to 30 minutes. Serve warm.

Pizzas and Flatbreads

Pavlov's Polenta Pizza

By Brian Hart

Jane's husband, Brian, is brilliant when it comes to food and recipes. He makes this polenta pizza and has every Esselstyn running for the kitchen like one of Pavlov's dogs when it comes out of the oven. Woof! Woof!

Prep time: 15 minutes • Cook time: 20 minutes • Serves 4 to 6

3 to 4 cups water (depending on your brand of polenta)

1 cup polenta

2 cups Easy 2 Make Pizza Sauce (page 161), Kale Pesto (page 229), or any E2-acceptable pizza sauce

2 cups fresh spinach

3 large tomatoes, sliced

1 cup cubed pineapple

½ cup roasted red peppers

2 garlic cloves, crushed

Other favorite pizza toppings: mushrooms, arugula, asparagus, or olives

⅓ cup nutritional yeast

Preheat the oven to 400°F. If using a pizza stone, sprinkle it with cornmeal; if using a pan, line it with parchment paper.

Bring the water to a boil. Add the polenta and whisk constantly until the mixture thickens and there are no lumps. (Instructions for preparing polenta vary from brand to brand—check the specific preparation instructions for yours.)

Pour the polenta onto the pizza stone or pan and flatten out into desired crust shape: round, square, mini, elephant, or fire-hydrant pizza. Prebake the polenta crust for 10 minutes.

Remove from the oven, add sauce and toppings, and sprinkle with the nutritional yeast. Return to oven and bake for 10 minutes. Slice into generous portions and serve warm.

Tip: To avoid a soggy pizza, precook the vegetables before placing them on the pizza.

J.R.'s Pizza and Flatbread Dough

By J.R. Rudberg

Firefighter extraordinaire J.R. attended a weeklong 2010 E2 Immersion Program in Austin. After he completed it, J.R. was empowered with a sense of control over food and is now a leader within the plant-strong healthy eating movement at Whole Foods Market. (J.R. is not only healthy on the inside now, but he has lost close to 100 pounds. Weigh to go, J.R.!)

Prep time: 5 minutes • Rising time: 20 minutes • Cook time: 5 to 15 minutes, depending on the thickness of dough • Serves 4 to 6

3 cups whole wheat flour, plus 1 cup for coating work surface and baking pans

1 packet active dry yeast

⅛ teaspoon salt (optional)

½ cup unsweetened applesauce

1¼ cups warm water

In a large bowl, blend together the flour, yeast, and salt, if using. Add the applesauce and water and mix in with a large spoon or fork until the mixture forms a ball of dough. Knead the dough ball on a flat working surface or right in the bowl until the dough tension increases. Add additional flour to your work surface and the outside of the dough if it is sticky, as needed. Cover the dough ball with a damp paper towel and set aside to rise for 10 minutes.

Preheat the oven to 400°F.

Divide dough into 4 to 6 equal-size hunks, depending on desired pizza or flatbread size. Knead each piece of dough into a firm ball, cover with a clean, damp cloth, and let rise for 10 minutes. Flatten out the dough by hand or with a rolling pin to the desired crust thickness, then, using a fork, poke numerous holes in it to limit crust bubbles. Bake on a flour-coated baking sheet, parchment paper–lined pan, or pizza stone.

The crusts can be baked with or without toppings—the time will vary depending on the thickness of the dough. Bake time is usually 5 minutes for a thin crust without toppings; 15 to 20 minutes for a thicker crust with toppings.

Easy 2 Make Pizza Sauce

By Jane Esselstyn

This fast and fresh pizza sauce will knock your homemade pizzas out of the park.

Prep time: 5 minutes (assuming Fast and Fresh Marinara is already prepared) • Cooking time: 10 minutes • Makes 2 cups sauce

2 cups Fast and Fresh Marinara Sauce (page 227)

1 tablespoon pure maple syrup

Fresh or dried oregano or other herbs of choice

Crushed red pepper flakes

Add 2 cups of the marinara sauce to a small pot; this allows for about ⅓ cup for each personal-size pizza. Add the maple syrup to the sauce in the pot. Cook the sauce over medium-low heat until it reduces and gets as thick as pizza sauce.

Taste the sauce at this stage and add the oregano, other herbs of choice, pepper flakes, or more maple syrup to taste. Use warm, or refrigerate until needed.

E2 Pizza Possibilities

Here are some recommended ingredient combinations for layering on top of J.R.'s Pizza Dough or any other dough that is E2 plant-strong approved.

The Asheville: Easy 2 Make Pizza Sauce (page 161), onions, artichokes, pineapple, and nutritional yeast

The Clevelander: Kale Pesto (page 229), mushrooms, and roasted red peppers

The Santa Ana: Plain Jane Hummus (page 221), caramelized onions, and olives

The Chattanooga: barbecue sauce, black-eyed peas, roasted corn, and scallions

The Santa Fe: Halle's Guacamole (page 225), green chilies, and red bell peppers

The St. Nick: Spinach-Artichoke Dip and Spread (page 224), grape tomatoes, and red pepper flakes

The Dragon Slayer: Arrabbiata Creamy Cashew Sauce (page 227), grilled zucchini slabs, grilled eggplant, grilled mushrooms, and fresh basil

The Book Group: Kale Pesto (page 229) or red sauce, arugula, tomato slices, and thin pear slices. Drizzle with balsamic glaze after baking.

Prepare J.R.'s Pizza and Flatbread Dough as directed (page 160). Prebake as many rounds of dough as needed. Build a pizza by layering any of the above options, or create your own. Bake in the oven for 5 minutes, or until all of the ingredients are warm and ready to be eaten!

E2 Flatbreads

Anything tastes good on a fresh, open-faced flatbread. Have a blast and let your imagination be your guide. We've thrown down some ideas to help get you started.

Try any of these recommended ingredient combinations:

The Bohemian: Hot Pink Hummus (page 221), edamame, grape tomato, and sprouts

The Gardener: Kale Butter 2.0 with Sweet Potato (page 218), fresh basil leaves, and tomato slices

The Austinite: OMG Walnut Sauce (page 216), broccoli, sprouts, and chopped bok choy

The Nottingham: Nottingham Sandwich Spread (page 224), tomato slices, and romaine lettuce

The Freudian Slip: nut butter and fresh peach slices

El Taco Plano: refried beans, avocado, salsa, and scallions

The Hanover: Guacamole Hummus (page 222), red bell peppers, and cucumber slices

The Ball Park: ketchup, mustard, relish, and a cooked, whole carrot

The Blake: mashed avocado, tamari-marinated tofu, pickled ginger, and shredded carrots

The Sunny Day: Fresh Anaheim and Edamame Spread (page 223), and tomato slices drizzled with Polly's Vinaigrette (page 213) or a balsamic glaze

The Hot Shot: Fire Hummus (page 222), orange and red bell pepper, fresh spinach, and jalapeños (if you dare)

Follow the instructions for J.R.'s Pizza and Flatbread Dough (page 160) to the stage where the dough is about to be flattened by hand or with a rolling pin. At this point, roll out the dough until it is less than ¼ inch thick. In a nonstick skillet over medium-high heat, grill the flattened dough until it rises in places, then flip to quickly cook the other side. Remove the flatbread from the pan and build an open-faced, plant-strong creation from the above options—or create your own. Serve immediately after preparing.

Maple Whole Wheat Bread Dough

By Jill Kolasinski

My wife, Jill, was first turned on to making bread by an Engine 2 potluck regular who brought mini, heart-shaped Engine 2 pizzas based on the recipe in my first book. When Jill asked her where she got the recipe for the crust, our friend told her about *Artisan Bread in Five Minutes a Day* by Jeff Hertzberg and Zoë François. The amazingly innovative aspect of this book is that it tells you how to make bread dough that can be refrigerated for up to two weeks! Then, whenever you want a fresh loaf, you just grab a ball of dough from the fridge and pop it in the oven. Jill bought the book and became so obsessed with baking bread that she took the book to bed with her every night and read it like a novel! Two years later, making bread dough has become a weekly routine. Kole and Sophie love helping Jill, and she has discovered other ways to use the refrigerated dough beyond just baking bread, such as for flatbread and pizza crusts. Having the refrigerated dough handy has become one of the tricks she depends on as a working mom to make sure our family has a hearty, nutritious meal every evening.

Prep time: 5 minutes • Rising time: 2 hours • Makes 2 loaves (you can halve or double this recipe)

1½ cups lukewarm water

1½ cups unsweetened almond milk, lukewarm

1½ tablespoons granulated yeast (2 packets) (Hodgson Mill makes a yeast especially for whole-grain breads)

1 tablespoon sea salt

½ cup pure maple syrup

6⅔ cups whole wheat flour (avoid pastry or graham flour)

In a large bowl stir together with a spoon the water, almond milk, yeast, sea salt, and maple syrup. Mix in the whole wheat flour; use your hands to mix in the last bits of flour into the wet ingredients—of course the kids love to do this! Let the dough sit at room temperature, until it rises and then flattens on the top, 2 to 3 hours.

Use the dough immediately to make any of the following options: a sandwich loaf, walnut-raisin loaf, flatbread, or pizza crust, or store it in a lidded plastic container, in the fridge for up to 5 days.

TO MAKE A SANDWICH LOAF

Preheat the oven to 350°F. Line a pizza stone with parchment paper if making a round loaf or lightly coat a 9 by 5-inch bread pan with nonstick spray if making a bread loaf.

Using a cantaloupe-size ball of the dough, sprinkle the top with flour. Sprinkle more flour on a cutting board, and plop the dough onto it. If the dough has been in the fridge, then it's best to shape the dough loaf and let it rise again for about 1½ hours.

Using a sharp, serrated knife, you can score the dough to make a letter or a pattern, if desired ("K" for Kole, "S" for Sophie, "M" for Mommy) while it rises. Slide the round loaf onto the pizza stone, or form and place in the prepared bread pan. Bake for 50 to 60 minutes.

TO MAKE WALNUT-RAISIN LOAF

Follow the directions for the round sandwich loaf, but before shaping the loaf, flatten the ball of the dough to a thickness of ½ inch. Sprinkle the flattened dough with ½ cup of chopped walnuts and ½ cup of raisins. Lightly knead and shape the round loaf with the nuts and raisins inside. Let rise for about 1 hour, if the dough is cold.

Bake at 350°F for 50 to 60 minutes.

TO MAKE FLATBREAD

Lightly spray a nonstick pan or cast-iron skillet, and preheat over low-medium heat.

Cut off a small ball of the refrigerated dough, about the size of an orange (you do not need to let it rise). Flatten the dough to a thickness of about ¼ inch, being careful not to tear it. Place it in the preheated pan, and cook, watching carefully to make sure it does not burn, until nicely browned on one side. Flip and brown the opposite side—just like a pancake. Repeat the procedure until all of the flatbread needed is prepared.

Tip: This flatbread is great with jam and almond or cashew butter. I also often serve it at dinner with broccoli and carrots on the side. Kids love to help flatten this bread!

TO MAKE PIZZA CRUST

Preheat the oven to 425°F. Prepare a pizza stone by sprinkling with cornmeal, or line a pizza pan with parchment paper.

Working similarly to the flatbread directions, cut off a bigger ball of dough about the size of a grapefruit. Flatten out the dough on a floured board to the desired thickness. Top it with tomato or pesto sauce and veggies.

For the kids, we make mini, individualized pizzas, topped with tomato sauce and sprinkled with nutritional yeast. Bake for about 20 minutes and serve.

Sandwiches

Rockin' Reuben on Rye

By Brian Hart

This was a shocker. My mom does not like tofu, ketchup, sauerkraut, pickles, rye bread, or tempeh. So when Brian made her a reuben on rye with tamari-roasted tempeh, tofu, ketchup-based Thousand Island dressing, and sauerkraut, she was shocked to find she not only liked it but ate four halves!

Prep time/cook time: 30 minutes • Makes 4 sandwiches

8 ounces tempeh
½ cup low-sodium tamari sauce
8 ounces silken tofu
⅓ cup ketchup
⅓ cup pickle relish
1 loaf rye bread
1 jar sauerkraut, your favorite
1 cup fresh spinach leaves

Preheat the oven to 350°F.

Slice the tempeh in half vertically and then horizontally, to make 4 thin, square patties. In a shallow dish, pour the tamari over the tempeh and marinate for 5 minutes, or more if time permits. Place the tempeh on a nonstick pan or on a pan lined with parchment paper and bake for 15 minutes.

In a bowl, mix together the tofu, ketchup, and relish until it looks like a tofu-based Thousand Island dressing.

Toast the rye bread to the desired crispiness. Spread with tofu-based Thousand Island dressing. Add a layer of sauerkraut, then tempeh, then spinach. Cut the sandwich in half and serve.

Day-After-Day Open-Faced Heirloom Tomato Sandwich

By Ann Esselstyn

Summer means heirloom tomatoes, and heirloom tomatoes mean open-faced tomato sandwiches—day after day after day. If you make these right, you can't have just one. You just can't.

Prep time/cook time: 10 minutes • Makes 6 open-faced sandwiches

6 slices rye bread
(Mestamacher or Brot)—
toast the dickens out of it!

1 cup Plain Jane Hummus
(page 221), or store-bought
hummus made with no
added oil or tahini

3 scallions, chopped

10 leaves fresh basil, chopped

3 large heirloom tomatoes, cut into
½-inch-thick slices

Balsamic glaze, preferably Isola
Classic Cream of Balsamic or the
Olive Tap Black Currant Balsamic
Vinegar

Toast the rye bread so that it is sturdy—2 to 3 times over. Seriously, two or three toasting cycles is what it takes in our toaster, but be careful not to burn it!

Spread with a layer of Plain Jane Hummus (page 221) or the store-bought hummus. Scatter the scallions and fresh basil on top of the hummus. Place thick tomato slab(s) on top of all. Drizzle with the balsamic glaze and serve.

Pepper Ridge Sandwiches

By Ann Esselstyn

Anyone is welcome to pitch in when our family makes more than one hundred of these sandwiches for our annual Christmas Carol party at my parents' house on Pepper Ridge Road. And every year they are devoured. People always ask, "What is the dressing used on these sandwiches?" There is no dressing! The dressing-like effect comes from the essence of roasted red bell peppers and the barbecued portobellos mixed with the avocado, spinach, and hummus.

Prep time/cook time: 50 minutes • Makes 4 to 6 sandwiches

3 red bell peppers

20 slices portobello
mushrooms

One 16-ounce jar barbe-
cue sauce, your favorite
(Bone Suckin' Sauce is our
favorite)

2 tablespoons balsamic vinegar

1 teaspoon dried oregano

1 teaspoon dried thyme

1 teaspoon dried rosemary

1 teaspoon dried basil

1 to 2 garlic cloves, minced

1 loaf Ezekiel 4:9 Sesame Sprouted
Whole Grain Bread

1 cup Plain Jane Hummus (page
221), or store-bought hummus
with no added oil or tahini

1 bunch scallions, chopped

One 6-ounce package baby
spinach

1 avocado, pitted, peeled, and sliced

Preheat the oven to 400°F.

Place the bell peppers in a pan and roast in the oven for 30 minutes, rotating the pan every 10 minutes.

Meanwhile, prepare the mushrooms. Place the mushroom slices on a parchment paper–lined sheet pan. Coat the mushrooms with barbecue sauce. Cook for 30 minutes in the oven, or until cooked through.

When the peppers are roasted, place them in a bowl and cover. As they steam and cool, the pepper skins will separate from the flesh. Peel the skins off the peppers and remove the stems and seeds. The peppers will weep their essence into the bowl—reserve this liquid in the bowl. Tear the peppers into strips.

Add the balsamic vinegar, oregano, thyme, rosemary, basil, and garlic to the pepper-filled bowl. If you prefer, toast the bread first.

To construct a sandwich, spread hummus on one piece of bread or toast. Sprinkle a thin layer of scallions over the hummus. Place a layer of barbe-cued portobellos on top of the scallions and hummus. Add a layer of roasted red peppers, a layer of spinach, and a layer of avocado. Place another piece of bread atop the stack. Slice the sandwich into halves or quarters and serve. Repeat the procedure to make the remaining sandwiches.

Tip: Try roasting your peppers Texas firefighter–style over a gas flame, over the grill, or in a hot cast-iron skillet until the skins blacken and puff away from the peppers.

ABCD Sandwich

By Jane Esselstyn

This sandwich is loaded with vitamin A from the carrots, vitamin B from the nutritional yeast, and vitamin C from the romaine lettuce. Eat this outside and you'll get your vitamin D, as well!

Prep time: 10 minutes • Makes 4 to 6 sandwiches

3 to 4 whole carrots, chopped
1 cup raw cashews
6 dates, pitted
1 tablespoon nutritional yeast
2 tablespoons water

1 loaf whole wheat bread, sliced
½ bunch scallions, chopped
1 head romaine lettuce, cleaned and chopped

In a food processor or high-speed blender, blend the carrots, cashews, dates, and nutritional yeast. Add water, as needed, until you reach the desired consistency; it should be similar to hummus.

Toast the bread. Spread a thick layer of the carrot-cashew mixture onto both slices of the toasted bread. Sprinkle 1 slice with the chopped scallions and a heap of the chopped romaine lettuce. Top with the other slice of toasted bread. Cut the sandwich in half, head outside, and enjoy.

Tip: If you prefer the sandwich less sweet, add fewer dates. If you like scallions, stir them into the spread as well as sprinkling them on top. Also, try red bell pepper and sprouts, or do what my nutritionally dense mother does and add steamed kale.

PBJB Burrito

Inspired by Elvis

The initials stand for Peanut Butter and Jelly Banana. Roll one up and you are ready to rock and roll! This one is in honor of the King himself.

Prep time: 3 minutes • Serves 1 to 2

    1 whole wheat burrito
    1 to 2 tablespoons peanut butter or other nut butter
    1 tablespoon jelly, preferably a no-sugar-added, fruit-only brand
    1 ripe banana

Spread a thin layer of peanut butter on the whole wheat burrito. Then spread with a layer of jelly. Place the banana on one side of the burrito, roll it all up, and eat!

The Mad Greek Gyro

By Jane Esselstyn

My two brothers, sister, and I could never pronounce these sandwiches correctly, but we sure could eat them: Gyros! Growing up in Cleveland, Ohio, Ted's, Jane's, Zeb's, and my favorite place to go was the Mad Greek restaurant at Cedar Lee Roads for "Jy-ros," "Ye-rohs," or "He-rohs." I have not tasted one made from meat in thirty years, but these plant-strong gyros remind me of the Mad Greek originals. Lip-smacking good!

Prep time: 40 minutes (varies per prepped ingredients) • Makes 6 gyros

Scary-Easy Seasoned Seitan (below), or use store-bought seitan

J.R.'s Flatbread (page 160) or any Engine 2–approved whole wheat bread or pita

Tzatziki Sauce (page 217)

1 tomato, sliced

1 cucumber, peeled and sliced

1 onion, sliced

Prepare the seitan (below) per instructions. Slice the seitan into thin strips.

Prepare the flatbread.

Prepare the Tzatziki Sauce.

To assemble the gyros, onto each flatbread layer place the seitan, tomato, cucumber, and onion, then cover with the Tzatziki Sauce. Fold the flatbread over and serve.

Tip: When making the flatbread, keep it thin, and do not overcook—keep it soft.

Scary-Easy Seasoned Seitan

By Jane Esselstyn

Do not be intimidated at the thought of preparing your own seitan. After you make this, your confidence will soar and nothing will get in your way. It is scary…scary easy! This seitan is perfect for the Mad Greek Gyro above.

Prep time/cook time: 45 minutes • Makes 6 to 8 gyros' worth of seitan

1¼ cups vegetable broth

1 tablespoon low-sodium tamari sauce

1 teaspoon minced fresh garlic

1 cup wheat gluten

1 teaspoon dried thyme

1 teaspoon dried rosemary

2 teaspoons dried oregano

1 teaspoon ground cumin

½ teaspoon dried sage

1 teaspoon onion powder

1 teaspoon garlic powder

2 tablespoons nutritional yeast

Preheat the oven to 375°F. Line a roasting pan with a layer of parchment paper.

In a large bowl, whisk together the broth, tamari, and garlic. In a separate bowl, mix together the wheat gluten, herbs and spices, and nutritional yeast. Combine the wet and dry ingredients. Hand mix and/or knead the ingredients until the dough has an elastic texture, about 3 minutes.

Flatten the dough in the lined roasting pan to a thickness of about ½ inch. Bake for 20 minutes, remove from the oven, baste with ¼ to ½ cup of the broth mixture, flip, return to the oven, and cook for 20 minutes more. Remove from the oven and let cool a bit before slicing.

Kale Bruschetta

By Jane Esselstyn

Kale is king, and as such the word deserves to be capitalized. From this moment on, Kale will be capitalized. It is that magnificent. This recipe is a huge hit at any party. Watch it vanish.

Prep time/cook time: 15 minutes • Makes 12 to 15 pieces bruschetta

   1 bunch Kale, leaves stripped of spines, spines discarded
   1 loaf whole-grain bread, sliced into 12 to 15 pieces
   ½ cup OMG Walnut Sauce (page 216)
   1 cup grape tomatoes, halved
   Balsamic glaze, preferably Isola Classic Cream of Balsamic

Place the leaves in a pot with an inch or so of water, cover, and boil over high heat for 4 to 5 minutes.

Toast as many pieces of bread as desired and place on a handsome platter. Spread the walnut sauce on the toasted bread. Layer the cooked Kale over the walnut sauce. Scatter the grape tomatoes over the Kale. Drizzle generously with the balsamic glaze and serve.

Warm Comfort Foods

Bad 2 the Bone Chili

By Brian Hart

Jane's husband, Brian, makes one bad-to-the-bone chili. And lucky for all of us, there is no muscle that used to be connected to any bone in this recipe.

Prep time/cook time: 30 minutes (plus 20 minutes for cooking dried lentils, if using) • Serves 10 to 12

One 12-ounce can lentils, drained and rinsed, or 1 cup dry lentils, cooked

1 large onion, julienned

2 red bell peppers, cut into long strips

4 celery stalks, chopped

2 medium yellow squash, cut into large cubes

2 medium zucchini, cut into large cubes

One 8-ounce package mushrooms, sliced

1 cup julienned carrots

One 28-ounce can whole, peeled tomatoes, with their juices

3 tablespoons chili powder

1 teaspoon ground cumin

One 40-ounce can kidney beans, drained and rinsed

2 to 3 tablespoons barbecue sauce, your favorite

1 to 2 tablespoons pure maple syrup

2 to 3 tablespoons salsa, your favorite

If using dried lentils, cook them using 2½ cups water to 1 cup lentils. Bring to a boil and simmer until the lentils are soft, about 20 minutes. Drain and set aside.

In a pot over medium-high heat, simmer together the onion, peppers, celery, squash, zucchini, mushrooms, and carrots.

Once all of the veggies are soft, decrease the heat to low. Add the whole, peeled tomatoes and their juices. Once in the pot, cut the whole tomatoes into pieces, using the edge of a spoon, a knife, or kitchen scissors. Add the chili powder and cumin. Increase the heat to medium, add the drained lentils, kidney beans, barbecue sauce, maple syrup, and salsa, and cook together for 2 to 3 minutes.

Simmer on low for 30 minutes. Brian says, "Taste it toward the end—add extra salsa, maple syrup, or chili powder according to your taste." Keep warm until ready to serve.

BBQ LOL (Lentil Oat Loaf)

By Ann Esselstyn

LOL suits this perfectly. Serve it up as the main dish with a big salad, or "fry" up leftovers the next day in an LOL sandwich. I especially dig the taste of the barbecue sauce on the top and bottom.

Prep time: 25 minutes • Cook time: 45 to 55 minutes • Makes 2 loaves; 8 servings

1½ cups red lentils
2½ cups water
1 large onion, chopped
One 8-ounce package mushrooms, chopped
4 garlic cloves, chopped
4 cups packed fresh spinach, chopped
One 15-ounce can diced tomatoes, with juices

1 teaspoon dried sage
1 teaspoon garlic powder
1 teaspoon Mrs. Dash Garlic & Herb seasoning blend, or similar spice blend
¼ teaspoon dried marjoram
½ cup chopped fresh cilantro or parsley, or as desired
2 cups old-fashioned rolled oats
1 to 1½ cups barbecue sauce or ketchup, your favorite

Preheat the oven to 375°F.

In a saucepan, bring the lentils to a boil in the water. Decrease the heat to low, cover, and simmer until the lentils are tender and most of the water is absorbed, 8 to 10 minutes. In the same saucepan, mash the lentils with the back of a spoon or a potato masher; don't worry, red lentils cook quickly and mash easily.

In a nonstick pan, cook the onions over medium heat, stirring constantly to avoid burning, until soft and translucent. Add the mushrooms and garlic and continue to cook over medium heat until soft. Add water or vegetable broth, if necessary, to keep the vegetables from sticking. Add the spinach, cover, and continue to cook over medium heat until the spinach wilts, 4 or 5 minutes.

Add the lentils to the onion-mushroom-spinach mixture and stir to combine. Add the diced tomatoes, sage, garlic powder, Mrs. Dash seasoning, marjoram, and cilantro and stir. Add the oats and stir it all again.

In the bottom of two 9 × 5-inch loaf pans, spread half of the barbecue sauce or ketchup. Add the lentil-oat mixture to the loaf pans, then spread the remaining barbecue sauce or ketchup in a generous layer on the tops.

Bake for 45 to 55 minutes until the barbecue glaze turns crispy on the edges. Let set for 10 to 15 minutes before cutting and serving—ideally until the next day!

Tip: The loaf is much easier to cut the next day.

Thank God It's Not Friday Restuffed Potatoes

By Ann Esselstyn

I first experienced restuffed potatoes at T.G.I. Friday's as a teenager with my whole family. Back in the day, they were stuffed with cheese and bacon bits and came with a heaping mound of sour cream on top. Boy, have things changed over the years. These are righteous on any day of the week, especially Fridays! Serve with steamed broccoli and a big salad.

Prep time/cook time: 90 minutes • Serves 6

6 medium Yukon Gold potatoes	Freshly ground black pepper
1 large, sweet onion, peeled and chopped	Pinch of cayenne pepper
5 garlic cloves, peeled	1 cup corn kernels, frozen or fresh
6 tablespoons nutritional yeast	½ cup scallions, chopped
½ cup unsalted vegetable broth	Paprika

Preheat the oven to 450°F.

Scrub the potatoes, prick with a fork, and bake for 1 hour. Spread the onion and garlic cloves out in a parchment paper–lined pan. Bake the onion and garlic for 20 minutes, or until browned but not burned.

Remove the onion and garlic from the oven and transfer to the bowl of a food processor. Process until smooth. After 1 hour, remove potatoes from the oven. Decrease the oven temperature to 350°F. Cut the potatoes in half. Scoop out the potato pulp, leaving enough to give the potato skin structure, and place the pulp into a large mixing bowl.

Arrange the empty skins in a handsome baking dish. Using an electric mixer, whip the hot potatoes, adding the onion mixture, nutritional yeast, and broth. Add a bit of extra broth if the potatoes seem dry—the desired texture is that of traditional mashed potatoes. Add the black pepper, cayenne, corn, and scallions, reserving some scallions for garnish, and fold into the mashed potatoes.

Spoon the mashed potatoes into the skins, sprinkle with paprika, and bake for 30 minutes. Sprinkle with the reserved scallions, and serve.

Hold on to Your Hat Steel-Cut Oats with Kale

By Ann Esselstyn

Oats and Kale! You'll never guess you are eating oats for dinner in this dish. If you've never made steel-cut oatmeal before, hold on to your hat, because this is one delicious dish. Seriously. Try this one on for size!

Prep time: 10 minutes • Cook time: 35 to 40 minutes • Serves 4

1 medium onion, chopped

2 to 3 garlic cloves, chopped

1 red bell pepper, chopped

4 cups (about 1 bunch) Kale, leaves stripped from stems and chopped

1 cup steel-cut oats

3 cups low-sodium or unsalted vegetable broth

3 tablespoons nutritional yeast

Hot sauce, your favorite

Freshly ground black pepper

In a nonstick pan over high heat, stir-fry the chopped onion until softened and beginning to brown, about 5 minutes.

Add a splash of water or vegetable broth if the pan is too dry. Add the garlic and bell pepper and cook for 1 or 2 minutes, adding a dash of liquid, if necessary. Add the Kale to the pan and cook about 3 minutes, until the Kale leaves reduce to about half their original size. Add the oats, broth, and nutritional yeast. Bring to a boil, cover, lower to a simmer, and cook for 25 minutes, or until all of the liquid is absorbed. Season with hot sauce and black pepper to taste.

Village Potato Pockets

By a small village of plant-strong chefs

There are many cooks behind this recipe. The original is adapted from Emma Christensen's food blog, *The Kitchn*, where she credits *Orangette*'s Chana Masala for the filling. And I credit Sarah Willis (Jane's sister-in-law) and Jane for making it an E2, plant-strong dish. It takes a village! You can change this recipe up a bit by using sweet potatoes instead of potatoes and Kale instead of spinach. Create your own version of a Village Pocket.

Prep time/cook time: 55 minutes • Makes 10 to 12 pockets

POCKETS

Follow the recipe for J.R.'s Pizza and Flatbread Dough (page 160), but *double the recipe* to make 12 instead of 6 pockets.

FILLING

1 onion, diced small

3 garlic cloves, minced

3 to 4 red potatoes, diced

1 teaspoon peeled and minced fresh ginger

2 teaspoons ground cumin

2 teaspoons garam masala

¼ teaspoon cayenne pepper (optional)

One 28-ounce can diced tomatoes, with their juices

1 cup peas, fresh or frozen

One 15-ounce can chickpeas, drained and rinsed

2 cups baby spinach leaves

To make the filling: In a deep pan over high heat, cook the diced onion and garlic until lightly browned. Decrease the heat to medium, add the potatoes, cover, and continue cooking until the potatoes soften on the outside. Keep an eye on the mixture, and add a tablespoon of water if needed.

Add the ginger, cumin, garam masala, and cayenne, if using, to the middle of the pan and heat until fragrant, about 30 seconds. Stir in the garlic, onions, and potatoes. Add the tomatoes and their juices and bring to a simmer. Cook, stirring occasionally, until the potatoes are completely soft and the sauce has reduced and thickened. Stir in the peas, chickpeas, and fresh spinach. Continue to cook over low heat, stirring, until the spinach wilts.

To make the pockets: Preheat the oven to 350°F. Line a sheet pan with parchment paper or use an aerated pizza pan (this is a cool pan to own if you do not have one).

On a floured work surface, working with one piece of dough at a time, roll out the dough into a round roughly ¼ inch thick. Place about ½ cup of filling onto the lower half of the flattened dough, leaving a ½-inch border around the edge. Fold the top of the dough over and pinch the edges closed as though you were making a calzone.

Transfer the filled pockets to the lined sheet pan. Repeat making pockets until all of the dough has been used; you should have 10 to 12 pockets. Arrange the pockets a few inches apart on the sheet pan. Bake for 12 minutes. Remove from the oven and serve warm.

Tip: I like dipping these pockets in a favorite dressing such as Jane's Dancing Dressing (page 214), Polly's Vinaigrette (page 213), or Ginger-Lime Dressing (page 216).

BBQ Seitan Grilling Kabobs

By Jane Esselstyn

When the *Forks Over Knives* production crew came by Fire Station 2 and filmed us sitting around the dinner table, our lieutenant, Scott Hembre, made this comment: "Barbecuing is a sport in Texas, and that's what guys do on weekends, they compete on barbecue teams to win contests."

Texans and firehouses across the country: Get ready to fire up your grills and let the barbecuing games begin!

Prep time/cook time: 40 minutes • Makes 6 to 8 shish kabobs

¾ cup vegetable broth

1 tablespoon low-sodium tamari sauce

1 teaspoon minced fresh garlic

1 cup wheat gluten

2 teaspoons smoked paprika

2 teaspoons onion powder

1 teaspoon garlic powder

2 tablespoons nutritional yeast

1 onion, chopped into large chunks

½ pineapple, sliced into large 1 by 2-inch square sections

1 red bell pepper, sliced into large 2-inch square sections

1 yellow bell pepper, sliced into large 2-inch square sections

One 8-ounce package white mushrooms

One 8-ounce container cherry tomatoes

Any other vegetables or fruits you want to spear on your kabob

1 cup barbecue or teriyaki sauce, tamari sauce, or your grilling flavor of choice

Preheat the oven to 375°F. Line a roasting pan with a layer of parchment paper.

In a small bowl, whisk together the broth, tamari, and garlic. In a separate bowl, mix together the wheat gluten, smoked paprika, onion powder, garlic powder, and nutritional yeast.

Combine the wet and dry ingredients. Hand mix and/or knead ingredients until there is an elastic texture to the dough, about 3 minutes. Flatten out the dough to a thickness of about ½ inch in the lined baking pan—this takes a bit of wrestling. Using a serrated knife, score the dough into a shish kabob–size (1 inch x 1 inch) grid, about 20 pieces. Bake for 15 minutes, remove from the oven, flip, and bake for 15 minutes more.

While the seitan is baking, slice the vegetables for the shish kabobs. Remove the seitan from the oven, coat with the barbecue sauce, return to the oven and bake for 15 minutes more. Remove the seitan from the oven and cut into cubes. Build the shish kabobs on skewers with the seitan cubes and sliced vegetables and fruit. Coat the shish kabobs with the barbecue sauce and grill until the veggies and fruits are bright and the sauce is browned. Serve warm.

Bubbles and Mash

By Jill Kolasinski

My wife, Jill, made these potato pancakes for the family one night out of the blue and we all loved them. I was enamored with their simplicity and asked her what in the world they were made of. She said they are derived from a peasant dish called Bubbles and Squeak, a traditional English dish made with left-over vegetables from a roast dinner. Similar dishes are made in Ireland and the Netherlands with Kale. We make it with onions, peas, corn, and Kale or spinach. You can make yours with whatever you've got!

Prep time: 45 minutes or 10 minutes if mashed potatoes are prepared •
Makes 8 to 10 potato pancakes

8 to 10 boiled potatoes	1 onion, diced
1 teaspoon ground pepper	½ teaspoon red chili flakes
1 teaspoon garlic powder	¼ cup frozen corn
1 teaspoon onion powder	¼ cup frozen peas
½ teaspoon salt (optional)	1 handful of chopped-up Kale or
3 tablespoons nutritional yeast	spinach

In a big bowl, smash the boiled potatoes into mashed potatoes, aka "mash." To the mash add the pepper, garlic powder, onion powder, salt (optional), and nutritional yeast and stir.

In a hot frying pan—so hot that a drop of water beads across the surface—cook the diced onion with the red chili flakes until brown and fragrant.

To the potato mash–filled bowl, add the cooked onion, corn, peas, and Kale or spinach and stir. Create palm-sized pancakes out of the mix.

In a nonstick frying pan on medium-low heat, place a hand-formed pancake of mash and veggie mix. Press the pancake down in the pan until it is about ¾ inch thick. Cook the patty until it is brown and crisp, then flip it. When you flip the patty, it may not stay together. If so, just push it back together again and continue browning the other side.

Serve with salsa or ketchup, or place in a bowl and ladle soup on top.

Tip: Using frozen veggies makes it fast and easy! Try frozen vegetable medleys, frozen corn, frozen chopped spinach, or frozen chopped Kale.

Cool Comfort Foods

Dr. Seuss Stacked Polenta

By Jane Esselstyn

Time and time again, this elegant, delicious recipe is a hit at our Engine 2 Immersion programs when Jane leads everyone in making his or her own Dr. Seuss Stacked Polenta!

Whenever Jane's kids stack all the ingredients in place and drizzle the star on the top, she is reminded of Dr. Seuss's Yertle the Turtle and Star-Bellied Sneetches.

Prep time/cook time: 50 minutes • Makes 12 to 15 stacks

1 to 2 large sweet potatoes, roughly the same girth as the polenta rounds

1 tube store-bought polenta

3 to 4 tomatoes, roughly the same girth as the polenta rounds

1 cup OMG Walnut Sauce (page 216)

1 bunch fresh cilantro or basil, your preference, stems removed

Juice of 1 lime or lemon, your preference

Balsamic glaze, preferably Isola Classic Cream of Balsamic, or similar brand

Preheat the oven to 350°F. Line two sheet pans with parchment paper or nonstick silicone mats.

Peel and slice the sweet potato into ⅓-inch-thick rounds; you will need 12 to 15. Place on the first lined sheet pan and bake for 30 to 40 minutes until cooked through.

Meanwhile, slice the polenta into ⅓-inch-thick rounds; you will need 12 to 15. Place on the second lined sheet pan and bake for 20 minutes.

Slice the tomatoes in thick, round slices. Make the walnut sauce.

In a small food processor make the cilantro-lime or basil-lemon topping. Combine the cilantro with the lime juice (or basil with the lemon juice) and pulse until coarsely chopped.

Place the baked polenta rounds on a handsome platter. Spread a thin layer of the walnut sauce over the top of each one. Stack a round of sweet potato on top of each coated polenta round. Spread a thin layer of walnut sauce on top of the sweet potato rounds. Place the tomato slices on top of the coated sweet potatoes. Dollop with the cilantro-lime topping (or basil-lemon topping). Drizzle the top, sides, and the plate with the balsamic glaze in a star pattern. Eat with a sharp knife and fork so the layers hold together!

Hunter-Gatherer Rainbow Quinoa

By Jane Esselstyn

This recipe is a hunter-and-gatherer blast. It uses up bits of fresh things you may have handy and will push you to combine things you don't always eat together. A clue to its name: Remember the grade-school anagram for the rainbow, *ROY G. BIV*? Red, Orange, Yellow, Green, Blue, Indigo, Violet! Ask your family or guests to name the foods that match each color of the rainbow.

Prep time: 15 minutes • Cook time: 20 minutes • Serves 4

2 cups quinoa, cooked

Red = ¼ cup seedless red grapes (or more if you prefer), halved

Orange = ¼ cup sliced carrot rounds

Orange = 6 dried apricots, chopped

Yellow = 1 fresh mango, cut into small cubes

Green = 1 avocado, pitted, peeled, and cut into cubes

Green = 3 scallions, thinly sliced

Green = 3 celery stalks, finely chopped

Blue = ¼ cup fresh blueberries (or more if you prefer)

Violet = purple onion, finely chopped

Violet = ¼ cup currants or raisins (raisins, of course, were purple grapes in their previous life)

Balsamic glaze, preferably Isola Classic Cream of Balsamic, or similar brand

¼ cup crushed raw cashews, toasted (optional)

In a large bowl, combine the quinoa with the colorful fruit and veggies. Serve on its own, or on a bed of arugula or baby greens.

Just before serving, drizzle with the balsamic glaze and sprinkle the cashews, if using, over the top.

Grilled Mango, Cilantro, and Black Beans over Rice

By Maria Steiner

No need to have meat or fake meat at your next BBQ. Grab a few of those beautiful mangoes and join the fun. If you don't have a mango, use pineapple!

Prep time: 40 minutes • Serves 4 to 6

2 cups brown rice, cooked

2 ripe mangoes, peeled, pitted, and sliced

Two 15-ounce cans black beans, drained and rinsed

2 cloves fresh garlic, minced

1 red bell pepper, seeded and chopped

¼ to ½ teaspoon crushed red pepper flakes

Juice of 1 lime

¼ to ½ cup chopped fresh cilantro

¼ teaspoon salt (optional)

1 jalapeño pepper, seeded and minced

½ cup chopped red onion

Pinch of ground cumin

Cook brown rice as directed. Grill the mango slices over medium-high heat, about 4 minutes on each side—they are best when tender but not mushy.

Remove the mango slices from the grill and chop into cubes. Transfer the mango to a mixing bowl and add the beans, garlic, pepper, pepper flakes, lime juice, cilantro, salt, jalapeño, red onion, and cumin. Refrigerate for at least 20 minutes.

Serve atop the brown rice.

Jane's Nori Rolls

By Jane Esselstyn

Every summer, all the Esselstyns converge at our family farm in New York state to rally around Ann's birthday in July. Typically there are eighteen of us working, swimming, biking, running, and playing all day long. By dinnertime, we are all famished. So that each one of us knows which night we are responsible for making dinner or doing the dishes (yuck), Jane makes a chart that hangs on the refrigerator door pairing family members with these chores. Every meal is outstanding, but the one we most look forward to is the one when Jane makes enough nori rolls for a small army and we successfully polish off each and every one!

Prep time: 40 minutes • Makes 4 nori rolls; 25 to 30 pieces

2 cups short-grain brown rice, cooked (this tends to be a stickier rice)

2 tablespoons brown-rice vinegar, if needed

1 package nori sheets (usually contains 7 to 10 sheets)

1 red bell pepper, seeded and cut lengthwise into thin strips

2 scallions, cut lengthwise into strips

½ cucumber, peeled, seeded, and cut lengthwise into thin strips

2 long carrots, peeled and cut lengthwise into long, thin strips

1 avocado, pitted, peeled, and cut lengthwise into thin slices

1 mango, peeled, pitted, and cut into strips

2 stalks bok choy, cut lengthwise into long strips

Wasabi powder

1 jar pickled ginger

½ cup low-sodium tamari sauce

Put the rice in a large bowl and stir. If the rice is not sticky, stir in brown-rice vinegar until the texture becomes sticky.

Place 1 sheet of nori flat on a dry surface. Spread about ½ cup or less of the rice on one-half of the flat sheet (like covering half of a tennis court). Place the vegetables of your choice horizontally in the middle of the flattened rice. Using both hands, and starting from the rice end, start rolling up the sheet. Carefully cover the vegetables and keep rolling. It will stick especially well if the rice is still a little warm. If your nori does not stick, try wetting it a little at the non-rice-covered end. Slice each roll with a sharp knife in ½-inch, medallion-style pieces.

Make the desired amount of wasabi paste by adding water to the wasabi powder as directed.

Serve nori pieces with little dishes of pickled ginger, wasabi, and low-sodium tamari to taste. Eat these just as they are, or dip in one or all of the little dishes.

Variation: Nori Noir! Try using black rice instead of brown for a sensational visual experience. The dark rounds look stunning with bright vegetables highlighting their centers!

Super Sushi Salad

By Rachael Laing

Many of us love veggie sushi but can't be bothered taking the time to make the rolls. This dish is equally delicious. Make a buffet of ingredients and let your guests pile their bowls high with wonderful vegetables.

Prep time: 20 minutes • Serves 4

2 cups short-grain brown rice, cooked

1 cup grated carrot

1 cucumber, peeled, seeded, and diced

2 avocados, pitted, peeled, and diced

4 cups fresh baby spinach

1 cup edamame, cooked and shelled

1 jar pickled ginger

4 nori sheets, or more if desired, cut into bite-size squares

Seasoned rice wine vinegar

Low-sodium tamari sauce

Wasabi powder

Optional: sautéed portobello mushrooms, bean sprouts, lightly cooked broccoli, grated daikon radish, or snow peas

Place the rice in individual bowls. Top with the grated carrot, cucumber, avocado, spinach, edamame, ginger, nori, and other desired vegetables. Drizzle on the rice vinegar, low-sodium tamari, and wasabi (made from the powder with water as directed) to taste. Serve.

Toby's Thai Spring Rolls

By Toby Rosenberg

Spring rolls are one of the mysterious foods I thought only existed in Thai or Asian restaurants. I've always loved ordering them and dipping them into yummy peanut sauce. Well, when Toby arrived at a potluck with her spring rolls, I was won over by this homemade version.

Prep time: 30 minutes • Makes 15 spring rolls

15 round rice wrappers, aka spring roll skin

1 cup julienned carrots

1 cup julienned cucumbers

1 cup julienned bok choy

1 cup fresh bean sprouts

1 bunch fresh cilantro, leaves only

10 to 20 large fresh basil leaves

2 cups romaine lettuce, chopped

One 6-ounce package thin brown rice noodles, cooked

Any other julienned veggies, of your choice

Soak one rice roll wrapper in a shallow plate of water (it doesn't need to be hot). When the wrapper is pliable, transfer it to a dry plate.

Meanwhile, place another wrapper in the shallow dish to soak. Open the soaked wrapper on the dry plate so it is round, like a face. Place the veggies and noodles in the middle, like a long wide nose in the middle of the face. Fold up the bottom (the chin). Fold down the top (the forehead). Fold one of the sides (the cheeks) over and roll the rest of the way. The wrapper sticks to itself.

Cut in half (or not). Serve with Toby's Peanut Dipping Sauce and Dressing (page 217).

Farro Dinner Salad

By Ann Esselstyn

If you've never had farro, it's high time you did. It's one of the "meatier" grains in texture and is extremely versatile in hot or cold dishes. This version of farro is served cold in a salad and is perfect for those hot summer nights. Serve on a bed of arugula or spring salad mix.

Prep time/cook time: 30 minutes • Serves 6 to 8

12 ounces farro, cooked

2 cups grape tomatoes, halved

1 cucumber, peeled, seeded, and chopped into small pieces

2 celery stalks, chopped into small pieces

1 red bell pepper, seeded and chopped into small pieces

1 bunch scallions, chopped

One 16-ounce package frozen corn kernels

1 mango, peeled, pitted, and cut into cubes

1 bunch fresh parsley, chopped (1 cup or more)

1 cup chopped fresh basil

½ cup chopped fresh mint

Zest and juice of 2 limes

Zest and segments of 1 orange

½ to 1 cup fresh orange juice (2 to 4 oranges)

In a large bowl mix the cooked farro with the grape tomatoes, cucumber, celery, red pepper, scallions, corn, mango, parsley, basil, and mint. Add the lime zest and lime juice to the bowl. Add the orange zest, orange segments, and orange juice.

Tacos! Burritos! Quesadillas!

Tucson Spicy Lentil Tacos

By Anne Minkus

In 2011 my mom, dad, sister Jane, Colin Campbell, and I gave a one-day "Healthy You" seminar in Tucson, Arizona. The night before the event we were invited to Anne Minkus's home to mingle with many of the plant-strong pillars of the community. Anne and the Healthy You Network are committed to mentoring plant-strong cooks and educating people about how to get healthy! We had an unforgettable weekend and dinner at Anne's home, with these Tucson Spicy Lentil Tacos leading the charge.

Prep time/cook time: 30 minutes • Makes 10 tacos

One 12-ounce can lentils, drained and rinsed, or 1 cup dry lentils, cooked

2 cups diced onions

2 tablespoons diced garlic

½ jalapeño pepper, diced

One 1.25-ounce package taco seasoning

2 cups vegetable broth

10 corn tortillas

Taco toppings: diced tomatoes, shredded lettuce, guacamole, peeled and shredded jicama, salsa

If using dried lentils, cook the lentils in 2½ cups of water to 1 cup lentils. Bring to a boil, then simmer until the lentils are soft, about 20 minutes.

Sauté the onions, garlic, and jalapeño in a couple of tablespoons of water. Add the cooked lentils and taco seasoning to the cooked onions-garlic-jalapeño mixture. Mix well to combine and add the broth. When the mixture begins to boil, reduce to a simmer, cover, and cook for 5 to 7 minutes.

Preheat the oven to 350°F. Hang the corn tortillas from an oven rack so that the two opposing sides of the tortillas hang down like wide, upside-down tacos. Bake the corn tortillas in the oven for 5 to 7 minutes.

Remove the warm corn tortillas from the rack and admire your new taco shells. Spoon the lentils into the tacos shells, then garnish, as desired, with the tomatoes, lettuce, jicama, guacamole, and salsa.

Variation: If desired, use romaine lettuce leaves as a wrap and do away with the taco shells.

Hawaiian BBQ Tacos

By Rebecca Corby with Green Island Catering, in good old Austin!

These barbecued tacos won "Tastiest and Most Creative Dish" the evening of our 2010 July Engine 2 potluck.

Prep time: 10 minutes • Makes 8 to 10 tacos

16 ounces tempeh, crumbled

2 tablespoons low-sodium tamari sauce

One 16-ounce jar barbecue sauce

10 corn tortillas

1 cup shredded lettuce

1 to 2 cups fresh pineapple, cut into cubes or bite-size pieces

1 bunch fresh cilantro, leaves and sprigs

Preheat the oven to 350°F.

Place the crumbled tempeh in a nonstick pan over medium heat. Add in the tamari and cook, stirring, until heated through. Add the barbecue sauce and stir until all of the tempeh is coated with the sauce.

Hang the corn tortillas from an oven rack so that the two opposing sides of the tortillas hang down like wide, upside-down tacos. Bake the corn tortillas in the oven for 5 to 7 minutes.

Remove the warm corn tortillas from the oven rack and admire your new taco shells. Scoop the tempeh onto the toasted corn tortillas. Add shredded lettuce, pineapple, and a sprig of fresh cilantro on top.

Variation: Instead of taco shells, use romaine lettuce leaves as the vehicle for transporting the barbecued tempeh and pineapple to your mouth.

8-3-1 Burritos

By Rip and Jane Esselstyn

A burro is a donkey that can carry just about any load heaped upon its back. *Burrito* is Spanish for "little donkey," and these hearty little burros can carry whatever you heap inside of them. This recipe contains eight veggies, three beans, and one grain, all wrapped together to keep you going all day and night. (8, 3, and 1 were the first three digits of our home phone number growing up. We still get a kick out of that.)

Prep time/cook time: 40 minutes • Makes 6 burritos

1 garlic clove, crushed and minced

1 onion, diced

4 ounces mushrooms, sliced

1 small zucchini, sliced

1 small yellow squash, sliced

1 red bell pepper, seeded and sliced

2 Kale leaves, stripped of spines and sliced

2 bok choy stalks, chopped

One 15-ounce can fat-free/ vegetarian refried beans (usually pinto beans)

One 15-ounce can black beans, drained and rinsed

One 15-ounce can black-eyed peas, drained and rinsed

2 cups cooked brown rice

½ cup salsa, your favorite

1 teaspoon ground cumin

½ teaspoon garlic salt (optional)

Crushed red pepper flakes

6 whole-grain burritos (also called wraps or tortillas), no added oil

Salsa, chopped romaine lettuce, cherry tomatoes, and Halle's Guacamole (page 225), for serving

Preheat the oven to 350°F. Line a sheet pan with parchment paper, or use a nonstick sheet pan.

In a large nonstick pan over high heat, cook the garlic, onion, mushrooms, zucchini, yellow squash, bell pepper, Kale, and bok choy until tender. Decrease the heat to medium, add the refried beans, black beans, black-eyed peas, and brown rice, and stir well to combine. Add the salsa, cumin, garlic salt, if using, and pepper flakes to taste and stir until evenly incorporated.

Scoop ½ cup or more of the mixture into the center area of a burrito wrap. Fold over the sides and place the burrito on the lined sheet pan—use a metal utensil to hold the sides down if they unfold. Continue assembling the burritos and placing them side by side on the sheet pan. For crispy burritos, bake uncovered; for softer burritos, cover with aluminum foil. Bake for 12 to 15 minutes until warmed and browned to your liking. Serve loaded up with Grape-Mango Salsa (page 243), chopped romaine, cherry tomatoes, and Halle's Guacamole (page 225).

ParmesaNO Collard Burritos

By Charlene Nolan

These are green packs of dynamite and arsenals of health. Prepare a ton of these. They make great hunger-fighting weaponry for lunch or dinner.

Prep time/cook time: 60 minutes • Makes 12 burritos

1 onion, chopped

2 bok choy stalks, chopped

1 large red bell pepper, seeded and diced

2 cups broccoli, chopped

1 teaspoon dried Italian seasoning

1 large sweet potato, cooked, peeled, and cut into cubes

½ teaspoon garlic powder

12 collard greens

One 32-ounce jar marinara sauce (or 4 cups Fast and Fresh Marinara Sauce, page 227)

½ cup raw cashews, finely ground

2 tablespoons nutritional yeast

¼ teaspoon garlic salt (optional)

2 tablespoons coarsely chopped fresh flat-leaf parsley

Preheat the oven to 350°F.

In a hot nonstick sauté pan, cook the onion until soft. Add the bok choy, bell pepper, broccoli, Italian seasoning, sweet potato, and garlic powder, stir to combine, and cook until warm.

Cut the main vein out of the collard greens about two-thirds of the way up (it should look like a "Pac-Man" with a nearly closed mouth after the stem is removed). Add 1 inch of water to a wide frying pan, and steam the collard greens one at a time for a few seconds on each side until they turn a nice bright green.

Stack the steamed collard leaves flat on the countertop while you cook the remaining leaves. Overlap 2 collard leaves, completely hiding the removed veined section and pairing up similar-size leaves.

Scoop the sweet potato–veggie filling onto the paired collard greens; the amount depends on the size of the collards. Roll up the greens like burritos (fold the bottom over the filling, then the left side, then the right, then roll whole thing over the top) and place in a shallow baking dish (flaps facing down).

Cover the collard burritos generously with the marinara sauce. Cover the whole dish with aluminum foil and bake for 30 minutes.

Meanwhile, make what the recipe author, Charlene, calls ParmesaNO by combining ground cashews, nutritional yeast, and garlic salt. After 30 minutes of cooking, uncover the collard burritos and sprinkle ParmesaNO over the whole dish. Continue baking for 10 minutes, uncovered, until the ParmesaNO turns golden brown. Garnish with fresh parsley and serve.

Tip: You can Tex-Mex this recipe up by changing the spices to cilantro, ground cumin, and ground coriander, and changing the sauce to salsa! Also, for a lighter dish, top with whole wheat panko bread crumbs and toasted sesame seeds instead of the cashews.

Black Bean and Sweet Potato Quesadillas

Inspired by Steve Hall

These quesadillas are a regular with the E2 plant-strong Hall family. They are simple to make and very satisfying. The Halls suggest eating them with a big green spinach salad and a red pepper for maximum iron absorption.

Prep time: 10 minutes • Cook time: 1 hour • Makes 4 large quesadillas

1 large sweet potato

1 cup cooked brown rice

1 cup salsa, plus more for serving

1 cup fresh spinach

1 cup black beans, drained and rinsed

8 ounces vegetarian, no-added-oil refried beans

¼ teaspoon onion powder

¼ teaspoon chili powder

¼ teaspoon ground cumin

6 to 8 whole wheat tortillas

1 jalapeño pepper, diced (optional)

Halle's Guacamole (page 225)

Preheat the oven to 375°F. Line a sheet pan with parchment paper.

An hour before you plan to eat, peel and quarter the sweet potato. Bake the sweet potato on the lined pan in the oven for 45 minutes to 1 hour, or until soft.

Meanwhile, prepare the rice on the stovetop or in a rice cooker. Remove the sweet potato from the oven and transfer to a mixing bowl. Mash the sweet potato with the salsa, rice, and fresh spinach. Place the sweet potato mash in a saucepan and mix in the black beans and refried beans and heat the mixture thoroughly over medium heat. Add the onion powder, chili powder, and cumin to taste, and stir to incorporate.

Place a tortilla in a nonstick frying pan over medium heat and slather the side facing up with the sweet potato–bean mixture. Add jalapeños, if using. Place a second whole wheat tortilla on top of the first. Press down on the top tortilla with a spatula, then cook in the pan for about 3 minutes. Flip the tortilla with the spatula and cook the opposite side for 3 minutes more. Voilà!

Cut into the desired number of sections. Serve topped with salsa and Halle's Guacamole or any variation thereof: bok guacamole, edamame guacamole, pea guacamole, etc.

Tip: Also try this using black-eyed peas or any other favorite beans instead of the black beans.

Pasta Creations

Summer Soba

By Jane Esselstyn

This is the perfect dinner on a clear summer night, sitting on the porch and watching the sunset: beautiful, colorful, and grounding. I often double or triple this recipe, as it is also a smash hit at a crowded potluck.

Prep time/cook time: 20 minutes • Serves 4

One 12-ounce package soba noodles (buckwheat, whole wheat, or any combination)

¼ cup rice vinegar

1 tablespoon, plus 2 teaspoons pure maple syrup

1 tablespoon low-sodium tamari sauce

½ red bell pepper, seeded and sliced

1 mango, pitted, peeled, and cut into cubes

1 avocado, pitted, peeled, and cut into cubes

½ cucumber, peeled, seeded, and cut into cubes

1 ounce (half a spice-size jar) sesame seeds

Cook the soba noodles according to the package directions. Drain the noodles, and rinse under cold running water immediately to stop them from cooking and sticking. Transfer to a large, beautiful bowl, or refrigerate until needed.

In a small bowl, combine the vinegar, maple syrup, and tamari. Taste-test the sauce by coating a veggie or a few noodles with it once it is mixed. Tweak the sauce with more of whatever you want: vinegar or maple syrup or tamari. Add the sauce to the noodles and toss thoroughly with your hands. Put the sliced and cubed fruit and vegetables around the edge of the noodles in the bowl.

In a pan over medium heat, toast the sesame seeds until browned and fragrant. Watch closely! Sprinkle the toasted sesame seeds over the entire dish. Serve with large salad tongs in order to grasp a little bit of each ingredient.

Dino Kale over Buckwheat Soba Noodles with Nutty Ginger Sauce

By Jane Esselstyn

The Nutty Ginger Sauce combined with the Dino Kale, red pepper, and soba noodles does a bang-up job of sticking to your ribs, yet doesn't leave you feeling like you have a bowling bowl in the pit of your stomach (as you do after eating a plate or two of cow meat).

Prep time/cook time: 15 minutes • Serves 6

> Nutty Ginger Sauce (page 230)
> Two 12-ounce packages buckwheat soba noodles
> 4 to 6 leaves dinosaur (or lacinato or *cavolo nero*) Kale, cut into fine strips
> 1 red bell pepper, seeded and diced

Prepare the Nutty Ginger Sauce.

Cook the soba noodles according to the package directions. Transfer the noodles to a bowl; pour Nutty Ginger Sauce over the noodles, and cover with a heap of the dino Kale strips. Garnish with the bell pepper and serve.

Tip: You can make soba noodles the day before if necessary. If you are not serving them immediately, rinse them under cool water until cool to the touch. This step prevents them from sticking. When it is time to make the dish, rinse the soba noodles under warm water, separating them gently with your fingers.

Roasted Harvest Pasta

By Katherine Lawrence

The sweetness of the roasted corn combines perfectly with the squash and sweet potato to offer a refreshing alternative to a regular old red sauce. This recipe is loaded with all kinds of immune-boosting ingredients, so step on up and get yourself some. No sniffles here!

Prep time/cook time: 50 minutes • Serves 4 to 6

> 2 cups butternut squash, peeled, seeded, and diced
> 2 cups sweet potato, peeled and diced
> 1 cup white onion, peeled and diced
> 5 garlic cloves, sliced
> 1 cup corn kernels
> 2 tablespoons, plus 1 cup vegetable broth
>
> ½ to 1 teaspoon freshly ground black pepper
> ½ to 1 teaspoon salt
> ½ teaspoon ground cinnamon
> ½ teaspoon dried sage
> 1 pound whole wheat penne or bow-tie pasta
> 1 cup unsweetened soy or other non-dairy milk

Preheat the oven to 400°F. Line a sheet pan with parchment paper or a nonstick silicone mat.

Place the squash, sweet potato, onion, garlic, corn, 2 tablespoons of broth, and the black pepper, salt, cinnamon, and sage in a large plastic Ziploc bag. Seal and shake until the ingredients are evenly mixed. Spread the vegetables out in a single layer on the lined sheet pan. Bake in the oven for 30 to 35 minutes, until the potatoes are tender.

Cook the pasta according to the package directions, then drain. Transfer the vegetables, soy milk (or non-dairy milk of choice), and 1 cup of broth into a blender and process until smooth. Pour the sauce over the cooked pasta and mix gently. Serve hot.

Pasta Pie

By Kreg Sterns

I think we all love a good pie, but how about a "pasta" pie? Well, you are in for a creative treat with this one! I met Kreg when he attended a Whole Foods Engine 2 Immersion seminar. When he's not cooking up a storm, Kreg's a sign artist and an indie rocker!

Prep time/cook time: 40 minutes • Makes one 9-inch pie

> 1 pound whole wheat capellini (angel hair pasta)
> One 8-ounce package mushrooms, sliced
> 1 cup peas, fresh or frozen
> ½ cup Kale Pesto (page 229)
> ½ cup Kreg's Cashew Cream or Spread (page 231)
> 1 cup whole wheat bread crumbs
> 2 tablespoons nutritional yeast

Cook the whole wheat pasta according to the package directions. Drain and let cool.

Sauté the mushrooms and peas in a nonstick pan over high heat. In a large bowl, combine the pasta, mushrooms, peas, Walnut Pesto (from *The Engine 2 Diet*) or Kale Pesto, and Kreg's Cashew Cream. Place the mixture in a 9-inch spring form pan or pie plate. In a small bowl, mix together the whole wheat bread crumbs and nutritional yeast. Dust the top of the pasta mixture with the bread crumb–nutritional yeast mixture. Bake for 20 minutes. Serve warm, cut into wedges.

Raise-the-Barn Butternut Squash–Vegetable Lasagna

By Brian Hart, God of Lasagna

This is the god of lasagnas, the lasagna from which the Raise-the-Roof Sweet Potato–Vegetable Lasagna in *The Engine 2 Diet* book was born. A few days before my cooking contest against the award-winning Austin Fire Department chef, Tim Lafuenta, at the new Whole Foods culinary center in Austin, I asked my brother-in-law Brian how I could take my lasagna into the stratosphere. He told me to "lose the beans," put in a sweet potato for "creaminess," and sprinkle the top with ground cashews as a finishing touch. The result was a masterpiece. This is the original masterpiece.

Prep time: 50 minutes • Cook time: 1 hour • Serves 12

1 butternut squash, halved, seeds and fiber removed

1 large onion, chopped

2 garlic cloves, minced

1 zucchini, cut into cubes

1 yellow squash, cut into cubes

One 8-ounce package mushrooms, sliced

1 red bell pepper, seeded and diced

2 bok choy stalks, chopped

One 16-ounce box frozen spinach

1 tablespoon fresh or dried oregano

1 tablespoon fresh or dried thyme

2 tablespoons chopped fresh basil, about 6 leaves

15 ounces firm tofu

½ cup walnuts

Two 8-ounce boxes whole wheat lasagna noodles

Three 25-ounce jars marinara sauce of choice (with no added oil) or Fast and Fresh Marinara Sauce (page 227)

1 to 2 tomatoes, thinly sliced

¼ to ½ cup nutritional yeast (optional)

⅓ cup cashews, ground or finely chopped (optional)

garnish with greens of choice (optional)

Preheat the oven to 375°F. Bake the butternut squash for about 40 minutes until soft, then peel the skin off and puree the pulp; you should have 2 to 3 cups. Set aside.

In a large sauté pan, cook the onion and garlic, then add the zucchini, yellow squash, mushrooms, bell pepper, bok choy, spinach, oregano, thyme, and basil and cook until soft. Set aside.

In a food processor, combine the tofu and walnuts and process until crumbly—this will create a ricotta-like layer. Set aside.

In the base of a 10 × 14-inch lasagna pan, spread a layer of butternut squash (you may not use all the puree you prepped). Place a layer of uncooked noodles on top of the butternut squash. Pour a layer of the marinara sauce on top of the noodles. Lay a thick layer of the cooked veggies on top of the red sauce. Place another layer of noodles on top of the veggies. Pour a layer of red sauce on top of the noodles. Spread the tofu-walnut mixture on top of the red sauce. Place another layer of noodles on top of the tofu mixture. Place a layer of red sauce on top of the noodles. And finally, place the thin tomato slices and a sprinkled layer of nutritional yeast or ground cashews, if using, on top of the last layer of red sauce.

Cover the lasagna with a sheet of aluminum foil. Bake for 50 minutes. Remove the foil during the last 10 minutes of the baking time. This lasagna is best if cooled for a bit before cutting and serving. Garnish with greens for an extra WOW factor!

Starry Night Vertical Lasagna

By Jane Esselstyn

Like Van Gogh's painting, this will become one of your masterpieces! It is one good-looking dish! Serve it when you need to win points or have virgin-plant-strong eaters over for dinner. It can be rolled up ahead of time, or have guests roll their own. This recipe has lots of directions, but a visual image of the finished product really helps keep it simple. Enjoy this warm or cold.

Prep time: 40 minutes • Cook time: 15 minutes (optional) • Serves 12 to 15

One 8-ounce box long whole wheat lasagna noodles
15 ounces tofu, light and firm
2 teaspoons fresh oregano, minced
2 teaspoons fresh thyme, minced
6 fresh basil leaves, minced
2 garlic cloves, minced
1 onion, diced
One 8-ounce package mushrooms, sliced
1 zucchini, diced
1 yellow summer squash, diced
1 red bell pepper, seeded and diced
Salt
Freshly ground black pepper
1 bunch Kale
1 cup Kale Pesto (page 229)
2 to 4 cups Fast and Fresh Marinara Sauce (page 227) or store-bought marinara with no oil added

Boil the lasagna noodles according to the package directions (these need to be long, not square, noodles) until done or just slightly al dente. Remove from the heat and drain. Balance the noodles around the edge of the pot so they will dry and not stick to each other, or wrap in plastic. Do *not* add oil to the lasagna noodles.

In a food processor, combine the tofu and 1 teaspoon each of the oregano and thyme and all of the basil, and pulse until it has the texture of ricotta. In a hot sauté pan, cook garlic, onion, and mushrooms, covering the pan with a lid for a moment or two to release some of the moisture from the onion. Decrease the heat to medium. Add the zucchini, yellow squash, and bell pepper. Cook until all of the vegetables are soft. Add the remaining oregano and thyme, and season with salt and pepper to taste.

In a large mixing bowl, combine the tofu-walnut mixture and the cooked veggies and mix well.

Meanwhile, strip and cook the bunch of Kale in an inch of water. Drain and set aside.

Now for the building of the Vertical Lasagna rolls: On a cutting board or a clean work surface, lay out one lasagna noodle. Spread a layer of the Kale Pesto uniformly along the length of the lasagna noodle. Lay a cooked Kale leaf (or two) flat on top of the pesto. Take a scoop of the tofu-veggie mixture and layer it ⅓ inch thick uniformly along the length of the lasagna noodle. Starting at one end of the coated noodle, begin rolling it up until you reach the end of the noodle. Place the rolled-up lasagna, vertically balanced on its flat surface, on a plate, serving dish, or lasagna pan if serving warm. Repeat until all of the noodles and/or filling are used up.

If placing on a platter, these will look like the beautiful swirls in Van Gogh's painting *Starry Night*. Pour warm marinara sauce generously over the tops and sides of the vertical lasagna rolls. If heating them up, cover with aluminum foil and place in a 350°F oven for 15 minutes. Serve warm with extra sauce and enjoy the compliments!

Variation: Use 2 sweet potatoes—cooked, peeled, and pureed—instead of Kale Pesto.

Kale Pesto Pasta

By Jane Esselstyn

Kale is king. Kale Pesto is queen.

Prep time: 15 minutes • Serves 8

> 16 ounces whole wheat pasta
> 2 cups fresh spring greens
> 1 cup Kale Pesto (page 229)

Cook the whole wheat pasta according to the package directions.

Lay a bed of spring greens in the bottom of eight bowls. On top of each bed of greens, add a serving of hot cooked pasta. Dollop 2 tablespoons of Kale Pesto on top of each bowl of pasta. Serve warm!

Burgers and Fries

Handstand Burgers

By Jeff Novick

Jeff Novick is a dietician, nutritionist, chef, comedian, and one of the leaders in the plant-strong revolution. If you ever get a chance to see him lecture, jump on it! You'll want to take this dynamic, knowledgeable, and cuddly man (who can do perfect handstands) home with you. Here is one of our favorite Novick burgers.

Prep time: 15 minutes • Makes 8 burgers

One 15-ounce can kidney beans (or 1½ cups cooked)

One 15-ounce can chickpeas (or 1½ cups cooked)

1 cup old-fashioned rolled oats

½ cup cooked brown rice

½ cup sweet potato, cooked, peeled, and mashed

¼ cup salsa

1 tablespoon curry powder

Other spices, such as garlic (optional)

Three to four 100 percent whole-grain buns

Condiments of choice: mustard, ketchup, relish, tomato slices, red onion slices, spinach, romaine, guacamole (optional)

Drain and rinse the beans and chickpeas. Transfer them to a bowl and mash with a fork or potato masher. Add the oats, rice, sweet potato, salsa, curry, and any other spice of choice and mix to combine well.

Divide the mixture into 8 or 10 equal-size pieces. Roll each piece into a ball, and then form into a patty. Transfer to a plate and let the patties air-dry in the refrigerator for 5 to 10 minutes.

Grill the patties in a nonstick pan over medium heat, or place under a broiler, until golden brown, about 3 minutes. The potato makes the burgers soft and quick cooking, so watch them when grilling. Flip and grill the opposite sides of the patties until golden brown. Serve either open-faced or on a whole-grain bun with all your favorite condiment options, a plate full of your favorite veggies, and a salad.

Tip: Make sure the bottom side of the burger is done before flipping so that the burger won't break into pieces.

Spicy Spinach and Black Bean Burgers

By Lindsay Nixon

One of my whole-food, plant-strong, no-added-oil kindred spirits is Lindsay Nixon, author of the highly popular and mightily delicious *Happy Herbivore* cookbooks. Lindsay is a dynamo. I am thrilled she has contributed to the recipe section.

Prep time: 10 minutes • Cook time: 10 to 12 minutes • Serves 4

One 15-ounce can black beans, drained and rinsed

1 tightly packed cup baby spinach, finely minced

2 tablespoons tomato paste or ketchup

1 tablespoon prepared yellow mustard

1 teaspoon garlic powder

1 teaspoon onion powder

½ teaspoon ground cumin

⅓ cup quick-cooking oats

Hot sauce, your favorite

3 to 4 whole wheat buns

Condiments of choice: mustard, ketchup, relish, tomato slices, red onion slices, spinach, romaine, guacamole (optional)

Preheat the oven to 400°F. Line a sheet pan with parchment paper.

In a large bowl, mash the black beans with a fork until no whole beans are left, but they are not total mush like refried beans. Add the minced spinach, tomato paste or ketchup, mustard, garlic powder, onion powder, cumin, oats, and hot sauce to taste (as much as you like) to the beans and stir until well combined.

Using your hands, shape 4 patties and place on the prepared pan. Bake for 10 to 12 minutes, until firm and lightly crisp. Carefully flip over and bake for 2 to 5 minutes more until lightly crisp on the outside.

Serve either open-faced or on a whole-grain bun with all your favorite condiment options, a plate full of your favorite veggies, and a salad.

Lentil Balls

By Vanessa Mirecki

These little lentil balls of love will spruce up any pasta dish. They also make for great appetizers dipped in salsa, hummus, or Kale Butter (page 218). Smoosh down to form a patty.

Prep time: 30 minutes • Cook time: 35 minutes • Makes 6 burgers

1 eggplant

1½ cups cooked lentils

¾ cup Grape-Nuts cereal

1 tablespoon chopped fresh flat-leaf parsley

¼ cup finely chopped onion

1 teaspoon dried oregano

1 tablespoon balsamic vinegar

Freshly ground black pepper

2 tablespoons chia seeds

Chipotle powder

Smoked paprika

Six 100 percent whole-grain buns

Condiments of choice: mustard, ketchup, relish, tomato slices, red onion slices, spinach, romaine, guacamole (optional)

Preheat the oven to 375°F. Line two sheet pans with parchment paper.

Place the eggplant on a sheet pan and bake in the oven for 20 to 40 minutes until soft. Remove the eggplant from the oven and peel off the skin (resembles a penguin removing its tuxedo, if it could). Puree the eggplant pulp with a fork or in a food processor until smooth.

Put the lentils, eggplant, cereal, parsley, onion, oregano, vinegar, and black pepper to taste in a large bowl. Add the chia seeds, chipotle powder, and smoked paprika to taste. Stir until uniformly mixed. Using your hands, form ping-pong-size balls or patties. Place the balls or patties on the lined sheet pans. Bake for about 35 minutes. Serve either open-faced or on a whole-grain bun with all your favorite condiment options, a plate full of your favorite veggies, and a salad.

P.S. Chorizo Patties

Inspiration from Laurie Buckley and Lindsay Nixon

Laurie Buckley, a passionate healthy eating specialist from the Plano, Texas, Whole Foods Market store, adapted this from Lindsay Nixon's recipe. She told me, "I like to use black quinoa because the end result looks frighteningly like beef. LOL." (FYI: "P.S." = plant-strong.)

Prep time: 30 minutes • Cook time: 5 minutes (plus 15 minutes if making quinoa from scratch) • Makes 4 to 6 burgers

1 cup black quinoa and 2 cups water, or 2 cups cooked quinoa

1 tablespoon red wine vinegar

2 tablespoons low-sodium tamari sauce

1 teaspoon granulated garlic

1¼ teaspoons granulated onion

1 teaspoon paprika

1 teaspoon dried oregano

1 tablespoon chili powder

Dash of ground cinnamon

2 to 3 tablespoons ketchup or tomato paste

1 tablespoon prepared yellow mustard

⅛ teaspoon liquid smoke (optional)

One 15-ounce can pinto beans, drained and rinsed

1 cup old-fashioned rolled oats

½ teaspoon garlic granules

½ teaspoon ground cumin

½ teaspoon chipotle powder

½ tablespoon chili powder

Hot sauce

¼ cup chopped fresh cilantro

Four to six 100 percent whole-grain buns

Condiments of choice: mustard, ketchup, relish, tomato slices, red onion slices, spinach, romaine, guacamole (optional)

If starting with uncooked quinoa, in a saucepan combine the water, quinoa, vinegar, tamari, granulated garlic, granulated onion, paprika, oregano, chili powder, cinnamon, ketchup, and mustard and bring to a boil. Reduce the heat to a simmer and cover until almost all the liquid is absorbed, 15 to 20 minutes, stirring occasionally. If desired, add ⅛ teaspoon of liquid smoke.

If starting with 2 cups of cooked quinoa, in a medium saucepan over medium-low heat, to the quinoa add the vinegar, tamari, granulated garlic, granulated onion, paprika, oregano, chili powder, cinnamon, ketchup, and mustard and stir to combine. Add liquid smoke, if desired. Remove from the heat and let cool for 15 minutes. Mix well.

In a food processor, pulse the pinto beans—do not puree; keep them chunky. Transfer to a bowl and add the rolled oats and quinoa mixture. Mix well. Add the garlic granules, cumin, chipotle powder, chili powder, hot sauce to taste, and cilantro. Shape the mixture into patties.

In a nonstick frying pan over medium-high heat, cook each side until browned. Serve either open-faced or on a whole-grain bun with all your favorite condiment options, a plate full of your favorite veggies, and a salad.

Lean, Mean, Green Split-Pea Burgers

By Dick DuBois

These are so tasty it is tempting to eat spoonfuls right out of the pan. Make a double batch and freeze the leftovers for an easy and convenient meal any time.

Prep and cook time: 1 hour • Cooling time: 30 minutes • Cook time: 10 minutes • Makes 12 burgers

1 onion, chopped

4 to 6 garlic cloves, chopped (about 2 tablespoons minced)

1 red bell pepper, seeded and chopped

One 8-ounce package mushrooms, sliced

3 cups vegetable broth

1 cup dry split peas

½ cup brown rice

1 teaspoon ground coriander

1 teaspoon ground cumin

1 teaspoon curry powder (garam masala is especially delicious)

1 cup plain, dry, whole-grain bread crumbs or whole wheat panko

¼ cup chia seeds

Freshly ground black pepper

Twelve 100 percent whole-grain buns

Condiments of choice: mustard, ketchup, relish, tomato slices, red onion slices, spinach, romaine, guacamole (optional)

In a casserole dish or pot, stir-fry the onion, garlic, bell pepper, and mushrooms for 4 minutes, or until softened. Add the broth, split peas, rice, coriander, cumin, and curry. Increase the heat to high and bring to a boil. Decrease the heat to low and simmer, covered, for 1 hour, or until the rice and peas are tender and the water has mostly evaporated. Check the pot after 30 minutes: If there is a lot of liquid, remove the lid and let cook, uncovered, for the second half hour.

Transfer the pea and rice mixture to a bowl and, using an immersion blender, blend until just combined—do not puree! If you do not have an immersion blender, mix with a few pulses in a food processor. Transfer the mixture to a bowl, add ¾ cup of the bread crumbs, the chia seeds (the chia help hold these together), and black pepper to taste to the rice and pea mixture and refrigerate for 30 minutes until it stiffens.

Shape the mixture into patties and coat each side with the remaining ¼ cup bread crumbs. Fry in a nonstick pan or, better, bake at 375°F for 10 minutes. After baking, turn and broil 2 minutes on each side or until the patties are just beginning to brown—be careful NOT to burn the patties. (Dick says he likes to broil his because it dries them out a little so they hold together better.)

Serve either open-faced or on whole-grain buns with all your favorite condiment options, a plate full of your favorite veggies, and a salad.

Tip: To make bread crumbs, place bread slices in a 200°F oven for about 15 minutes, or until dried out. Then transfer to a food processor and blend.

Beer-Battered Onion Rings

By Jane Esselstyn and the Roofer

Jane's roof had sprung a leak, so she called the local roofer. After he finished fixing the leak, he mentioned that he knew all about the Esselstyns because he had read *The Engine 2 Diet*! Then he asked Jane what she was serving for dinner. When Jane said onion rings, he asked if she dipped them in a beer batter. Jane said she wasn't planning on it but she loved the idea and would break out the beer. You never know where the next great idea will come from!

Prep time: 15 minutes • Cook time: 30 minutes • Makes 15 to 20 rings

1 onion, sweet or Vidalia
½ cup white whole wheat flour
¾ cup beer
½ cup whole wheat bread crumbs
½ cup corn flake crumbs (available in a canister—not from the cereal)

1 teaspoon onion powder
1 teaspoon garlic powder
1 teaspoon salt (optional)
1 teaspoon Cajun seasoning
2 tablespoons nutritional yeast

Preheat the oven to 400°F. Line a sheet pan with parchment paper or a nonstick silicone mat, or use a nonstick sheet pan.

Cut the onions crosswise into ½-inch-thick rings. Pop the little onion rings out of the bigger ones—these are some of my favorites because they end up being so crunchy.

In a large bowl, combine the whole wheat flour and beer and stir. In a separate bowl, combine the bread crumbs, corn flake crumbs, onion powder, garlic powder, salt, Cajun seasoning, and nutritional yeast. Follow the next set of instructions in assembly line fashion—if possible, it's nice to have one person at each of the bowl stations.

Dip the onion rings into the beer batter, coating all the surfaces well. Place the batter-coated rings one at a time into the bread-crumb bowl one at a time and toss crumbs all over the rings. Place coated and crumb-covered onion rings into the pan. Bake at 400°F for 15 minutes, then flip the rings and bake 15 minutes on the opposite sides for crispy rings, or less than 15 minutes for softer rings. Remove from the oven and enjoy with ketchup or other dipping sauces.

Eggplant Fries

By Jane Esselstyn

I have never liked eggplant as much as other people—there's something about its consistency and chewiness that doesn't appeal to me. Yet these eggplant fries defy all that; they are the exception to the rule for anyone who feels the way I do about the purple plant.

Prep time: 15 minutes • Cook time: 30 minutes • Makes about 30 fries (varies with size of eggplant used)

1 medium eggplant	2 tablespoons nutritional yeast
2 cups almond milk	1 teaspoon salt (optional)
2 teaspoons flaxseed meal	1 teaspoon onion powder
1 teaspoon apple cider vinegar	1 teaspoon garlic powder
2 cups whole wheat bread crumbs	

Preheat the oven to 400°F. Line a sheet pan with parchment paper or a nonstick silicone mat, or use a nonstick sheet pan and set aside.

Peel the eggplant and cut lengthwise into strips about the thickness of chopsticks and as long as you like.

In a medium bowl, combine the almond milk, flaxseed, and vinegar.

In a separate bowl, mix the whole wheat bread crumbs, nutritional yeast, salt, if using, onion powder, and garlic powder. Follow the next set of instructions in assembly line fashion—it is nice to have one person at each of the bowl stations.

Dip the eggplant strips into the almond milk mixture, coating all surfaces well. Place the coated eggplant strips into the bread-crumb bowl and toss crumbs all over the strips. Place the coated and crumb-covered eggplant strips onto the pan. Bake for 15 to 20 minutes, then flip eggplant strips and bake for 15 to 20 minutes on the opposite sides. Remove from the oven and enjoy with ketchup or other dipping sauces.

Variation: If you are not a fan of eggplant, make Zucchini Fries by substituting zucchini for the eggplant and following the same recipe instructions.

Carrot Fries

By Lindsay Nixon

This is a whole 'nother twist on healthy fries—thanks, Bugs Bunny!

Prep time: 10 minutes • Cook time: 30 minutes • Serves 6

> 1 pound baby carrots
> Onion powder (granulated, not flour-like)
> Salt (optional)
> Freshly ground black pepper

Preheat the oven to 400°F. Line a baking sheet with parchment paper and set aside.

Cut the baby carrots in half lengthwise (if you come across any large ones, cut them in half again). Place carrots in a colander and rinse under cold running water, shaking to remove excess water, but don't dry them completely.

Sprinkle the carrots generously with onion powder, salt, if using, and pepper, then toss with your hands to distribute the seasonings. Add more seasonings to taste and repeat until the carrots are well coated.

Transfer the carrots to your prepared baking sheet. Make sure there is no overlap, and use your fingers to reposition the carrots as necessary. Bake for 20 to 35 minutes until the carrots are fork-tender. Serve with your favorite ketchup or dip.

Tip: Try this recipe with zucchini, yellow squash, or parsnips.

Cleveland Tofu Fries and "Fish" Sticks

By Jane Esselstyn

One of the things I remember while growing up was gobbling up fish sticks hot out of the oven, dipped in ketchup. These are delicious and take me back to our kitchen in Cleveland, Ohio. Feed these to your kids instead of the "real" thing.

Prep time: 15 minutes • Cook time: 30 minutes • Serves 4 to 6

One package firm tofu, drained (for 24 hours if possible)

1 to 2 cups unsweetened almond milk

2 cups whole wheat bread crumbs

2 teaspoons onion powder

1 teaspoon garlic salt

2 to 3 tablespoons nutritional yeast

Kelp flakes (optional; for adding a fishy flavor)

Salt (optional)

Preheat the oven to 400°F. Line a baking sheet with parchment paper or a nonstick silicone liner and set aside.

Cut the drained tofu into fries, little fish shapes, or whatever shape you desire.

Pour the almond milk into a bowl.

In a separate bowl, combine the whole wheat bread crumbs, onion powder, garlic salt, and nutritional yeast.

Follow the next set of instructions in assembly line fashion—as always, it's nice to have one person at each of the bowl stations.

Dip the tofu into the almond milk, coating all surfaces well. Place the coated tofu into the bread-crumb bowl and toss the crumbs all over the strips. Place the coated and crumb-covered tofu onto the lined pan. Bake for 15 minutes, flip the tofu, and bake for 15 minutes on the opposite sides.

Remove from the oven, sprinkle with the Kale flakes and/or salt, if using, and enjoy with ketchup or other dipping sauces.

Crispy Polenta Strips

By Jane Esselstyn

Load these spicy little numbers onto your plate to complement any plant-strong burger. They are a crisp and fiery kick in the pants.

Prep time: 15 minutes • Cook time: 30 minutes • Serves 6 to 8

1 store-bought tube polenta

1 to 2 cups almond milk

2 cups corn flake crumbs (from a canister, not from your old cereal boxes!)

2 teaspoons garlic powder or garlic salt

2 tablespoons nutritional yeast

¼ cup taco seasoning or Southwestern spice

2 shakes crushed red pepper flakes

Hot sauce or ketchup, your favorite

Preheat the oven to 400°F. Line a baking sheet with parchment paper and set aside.

Cut the polenta lengthwise into fry-size strips.

Pour the almond milk into a bowl.

In a separate bowl, combine the corn flake crumbs, garlic powder or garlic salt, nutritional yeast, Southwestern spice, and pepper flakes.

Follow the next set of instructions in assembly line fashion—as always, it's nice to have one person at each of the bowl stations.

Dip the polenta strips into the almond milk, coating all surfaces well. Place the polenta strips into the corn flake crumb bowl and toss the crumbs all over the polenta. Place coated and crumb-covered polenta strips onto the lined pan.

Bake for 15 minutes, flip polenta strips, and bake for 15 or more minutes on the opposite sides for crispy strips.

Remove from the oven and enjoy with ketchup or other dipping sauces.

Dressings and Dips

Polly's Vinaigrette

By Polly LaBarre

This salad dressing was created by the one and only Polly LaBarre, the love of my brother, Zeb. They fit together like rice and beans. In fact, they fit together like the below ingredients to form a refreshingly superb, no-nonsense dressing.

Prep time: 5 minutes • Makes ½ cup vinaigrette

2 large garlic cloves, crushed and minced

¼ cup Olive Tap Black Currant Balsamic Vinegar

1 teaspoon Dijon mustard

2 teaspoons hummus

1 teaspoon dried thyme or chopped fresh thyme leaves

1 twist freshly ground black pepper

1 twist freshly ground sea salt

Ready a lidded jar or container. Crush the big garlic cloves into the jar.

Add the vinegar to the jar or container. Add the Dijon, hummus, thyme, black pepper, and salt. Close the jar and shake vigorously to emulsify (it's a mini arm workout). Taste and adjust the seasonings as needed.

Tip 1: Double this recipe so you'll have more on hand when needed!

Tip 2: Polly strongly recommends the Olive Tap brand vinegars because they are creamy and less sharp than conventional balsamics—totally worth it! Find them at a store near you or online (www.OliveTap.com). It will revolutionize the way you eat salads.

Balsamic-Berry Dressing

Inspired by Jill Nussinow, aka the Veggie Queen

The Veggie Queen was the first person to send Austin's Engine 2 firefighters a copy of her cookbook after an article about us appeared in the *New York Times* back in early 2006. We loved making her recipes because, well, she's the queen of veggies!

Prep time: 5 minutes • Makes about 1 cup dressing

1 cup ripe berries, your choice

2 to 3 tablespoons balsamic vinegar

2 teaspoons pure maple syrup

2 teaspoons mustard, your choice

Freshly ground black pepper

Place all of the ingredients into a blender or food processor and blend well. Serve over a salad or any other veggies.

Every Single Day Miso Dressing

By Adrienne Hart

Go ahead and double or triple this recipe so you can eat it every single day of the week! It's that good.

Prep time: 5 minutes • Makes about ½ cup dressing

2 tablespoons yellow miso
2 teaspoons peeled and grated fresh ginger
2 tablespoons pure maple syrup
1 tablespoon rice vinegar
3 tablespoons water

Whisk together all of the ingredients. Serve over salad or cooked greens.

Jane's Dancing Dressing

By Jane Esselstyn

This dressing dances with the depth of vinegar, the adventure of mustard, the sweet kiss of maple syrup, and the refreshing zing of lemon. Put it on your dance card tonight and watch your salad swing!

Prep time: 2 minutes • Makes almost ½ cup dressing

3 tablespoons balsamic vinegar
2 tablespoons mustard, your choice
1 tablespoon pure maple syrup
1 tablespoon fresh lemon juice
Chopped fresh dill (optional)

Combine the vinegar, mustard, maple syrup, and lemon juice in a bowl and whisk until uniformly mixed. Add the chopped fresh dill, if using. Serve over salad or cooked greens.

Super-Duper Dressing

*Inspired by acai superfood dressing from the
Colorado Springs Whole Foods Market*

This super-duper dressing throws a superhero cape of flavor over any salad. Enjoy it, you superheroes of health!

Prep time: 5 minutes • Makes 1¼ cups dressing

1 cup acai juice (made from frozen acai concentrate)

2 tablespoons apple cider vinegar

½ teaspoon minced garlic

½ teaspoon salt

½ teaspoon freshly ground black pepper

Pinch of cayenne pepper

½ cup raw cashews, soaked overnight

1 tablespoon pure maple syrup or fruit puree made from soaked apricots or dates

Make the acai juice from frozen concentrate as directed. Blend all of the ingredients in a food processor or high-speed blender until smooth. Pour over salad, toss, and serve.

Garlicky Tahini Dressing

Inspired by a similar dressing at the Princeton Whole Foods Market

Whole Foods Market is supporting its healthy eating campaign with Wellness Clubs inside the stores, where people can take cooking classes, listen to lectures, and join a community that values healthy living. I've been to all five brick-and-mortar Wellness Clubs throughout the United States, and they are all terrific.

I discovered this dressing after spending two days at the Princeton, New Jersey, club and I was utterly blown away. Now it's your turn to whip it up and blow yourself away!

Prep time: 5 minutes • Makes 2½ cups dressing

1 cup tahini

½ cup rice vinegar

3 tablespoons pure maple syrup

½ cup water

2 tablespoons low-sodium tamari sauce

2 tablespoons nutritional yeast

1 heaping tablespoon minced fresh garlic

2 scallions, thinly sliced

Combine all of the ingredients, except for the scallions, in a food processor and puree until smooth. Stir in the scallions, and serve over salad or greens.

Ginger-Lime Dressing

By Mary Schleicher

Mary Schleicher is a librarian who knows how to find a good thing without using the Dewey Decimal System! This versatile dressing works equally well over a green salad, vegetables, other greens, and/or grains. Some even find it tasty over a bowl of fruit, oats, or cereal.

Prep time: 10 minutes • Makes 1 cup dressing

½ cup silken tofu (about ½ of 12-ounce package)
2 teaspoons peeled and grated fresh ginger
Juice of 1½ limes
4 teaspoons pure maple syrup
2 teaspoons sesame seeds, toasted

Blend all of the ingredients in a food processor, scraping down the sides at least once. Blend again, and serve.

OMG Walnut Sauce

By Ann Esselstyn

This sauce is the gold standard against which all other sauces are measured and compared. This sauce got us eating Kale by the bushel. This is a sauce that you will love. For those of you who have yet to develop an appreciation for the taste of Kale, arugula, mustard greens, collard greens, beet greens, or anise, this dressing will help make those cruciferous green leafy vegetables go down. Also try it on the Austinite Flatbread (page 163) for lunch.

Prep time: 5 minutes • Makes about 1½ cups sauce

1 cup walnuts
2 to 4 garlic cloves
1 tablespoon low-sodium tamari sauce
¼ to ½ cup water, for desired consistency

Combine the walnuts, garlic, and tamari in a food processor and blend, adding water until the desired texture is reached (¼ to ½ cup); use more water for a thinner dressing, less water for a thicker dip (this is an amazing stage; the mixture suddenly turns white and creamy!).

Serve over Kale, greens, salads, grains, or veggies, or use as a spread in sandwiches or as a topping on pizza.

Tip: Create an amazing combination by mixing two favorites: Every Single Day Miso Dressing (page 214) and OMG Walnut Sauce. Boom! You'll love it!

Toby's Peanut Dipping Sauce and Dressing

By Toby Rosenberg

Some things really are meant to go together: yin and yang, night and day, Batman and Robin, and this sauce and Toby's Thai Spring Rolls (page 187).

Prep time: 8 minutes • Makes 1½ cups sauce

1 large garlic clove, peeled
One 1-inch chunk fresh ginger, peeled and grated
⅓ to ½ cup water
½ cup natural peanut butter or almond butter
2 tablespoons sweet white miso

1 tablespoon low-sodium tamari sauce
3 tablespoons fresh lime juice or lemon juice
Cayenne pepper (optional)
1 to 2 tablespoons pure maple syrup

Blend all of the ingredients together in a food processor or high-speed blender for creamy consistency, and serve.

Tzatziki Sauce

By Valerie Lee

This sauce is a healthy version of the similar sauce that can turn an everyday gyro into a deity to be worshipped at the altar of your mouth. You can find the Mad Greek Gyro recipe on page 171.

Prep time: 10 minutes • Makes 2 cups sauce

One 12-ounce box silken tofu
2 garlic cloves
Juice of 1 lemon
2 teaspoons dried dill or 1½ tablespoons chopped fresh dill
½ cucumber, peeled and grated
Freshly ground black pepper

Place the tofu in a food processor or high-speed blender along with the garlic, lemon juice, dill, and cucumber and blend until creamy. Season with pepper to taste.

Kale Butter 2.0 with Sweet Potato

By Dani Little

This incarnation of Kale butter is from Dani Little, the Engine 2 program director and nutritionist. According to Dani, "This makes a Kale lover outta anyone! It also supports absorption of iron. The sweet potato contributes vitamin C, which is needed to support non-heme iron absorption. Woo!" Try this on the Gardener Flatbread (page 163) for lunch.

Prep time: 10 minutes • Makes 2 to 3 cups Kale butter

> 1 bunch Kale, leaves stripped of spines, spines discarded
> ½ cup walnuts
> 1 sweet potato, baked and peeled
> Salt

Steam the Kale for about 5 minutes until tender, and drain.

Toast the walnuts until fragrant.

Place the Kale, walnuts, and precooked sweet potato in a food processor or high-speed blender and blend until smooth. Add water as needed to achieve the desired texture, about ½ cup. Add salt to taste, if desired.

Serve on anything, spread on everything, and eat often.

Mommy's Mushroom Gravy

By Ann Esselstyn

I love this best on No-Moo-Here Mashed Potatoes (page 154) or over baked potatoes, rice, millet, polenta, Lynn's Meatloaf (on page 204 of *The Engine 2 Diet*), burgers (outside the bun), or even just toast!

Prep time/cook time: 20 minutes • Makes 4 cups gravy

1 onion, chopped	2 tablespoons whole wheat flour
2 to 3 garlic cloves, minced	1 tablespoon low-sodium tamari
12 ounces mushrooms, sliced	sauce
2 cups vegetable broth	2 tablespoons sherry (optional)
1 tablespoon miso	Freshly ground black pepper

Stir-fry the onion over medium-high heat; add a splash of water or broth if it starts to burn.

Allow the onion to brown a little, scrape the pan, add a splash of liquid, and let it brown some more, but watch carefully so it doesn't burn.

Add the garlic and sliced mushrooms and continue cooking until the mushrooms are soft.

Add a bit of vegetable broth or water, as needed, to keep the mixture from burning.

Add 1 cup of the broth and stir.

Add the miso, whole wheat flour, and tamari sauce to the remaining cup of broth and stir until dissolved. Add the dissolved miso and flour mixture to the pan along with the 2 tablespoons of sherry, if using. Continue cooking until the gravy thickens to your liking.

Season with pepper to taste. Serve warm.

Tip: If you have time, roast the onions, garlic, and mushrooms in a 400°F oven for 15 minutes instead of stir-frying them.

Hummus and Spreads

Hot Pink Hummus

By Jane and Zeb Esselstyn Hart

This is how Jane's son, Zeb (named after his uncle), makes his favorite hummus. He crushes the garlic's protective skin, explodes the bulb through a press, cranks the can opener, blasts the beans clean, reams the lemon for its juice, combines and grinds it all in the food processor, then tosses in a beet grenade and watches the white mixture bleed into hot pink! So exciting! Try this on the Bohemian Flatbread (page 163) for lunch or the Santa Ana Pizza (page 162) for dinner.

Prep time: 10 minutes • Makes 1½ to 2 cups hummus

One 15-ounce can chickpeas, drained and rinsed
2 garlic cloves, crushed
Juice of ½ lemon
1 tablespoon tahini (optional)
½ teaspoon salt
1 beet, cooked and peeled

In a food processor, combine the chickpeas, garlic, lemon juice, tahini, and salt (if using) and pulse until well mixed. Add water to thin as needed to achieve the desired texture, and the beet for color. Serve. Refrigerate leftovers.

Variation: For Plain Jane Hummus, leave out the beet!

Great Green Spinach Hummus

By Ann Esselstyn

This is beautiful, green, and quick to make! Use more or less of the ingredients you like—especially cilantro, lemon, or garlic.

Prep time: 10 minutes • Makes 1¾ cups hummus

2 garlic cloves
One 15-ounce can chickpeas, drained and rinsed
¼ teaspoon ground cumin
2 tablespoons nutritional yeast (heaping ones, if you wish)
¼ cup fresh orange juice
Zest of 1 lemon
3 tablespoons fresh lemon juice
¼ to ½ cup fresh cilantro leaves, as desired
1 cup fresh spinach
2 scallions, chopped

Place all of the ingredients in a food processor and blend until smooth.

Serve with toasted pita bread and raw vegetables or use as a sandwich spread.

Tip: Try using this as a base for salad dressing by adding balsamic vinegar!

Fire Hummus

By Rachel Safran

This is flamin' good stuff! Rachel, the prepared-food team leader at the Henderson Whole Foods Market store in Las Vegas, took it upon herself to help Jane and me develop this "fire hummus" recipe. Try this on the Hot Shot Flatbread (page 163) for lunch.

Prep time: 8 minutes • Makes 2 cups hummus

2 dried chipotle peppers, reconstituted in water overnight, chopped

3 tablespoons tahini

3 tablespoons low-sodium tamari sauce

One 15-ounce can chickpeas, drained and rinsed

2 teaspoons ground cumin

4 garlic cloves

½ red bell pepper, seeded and chopped

3 tablespoons fresh lemon juice

4 to 5 tablespoons of the water used to reconstitute the chipotles

Place the dried chipotles in a bowl with enough warm water to cover the peppers and soak overnight.

The next day, remove the chipotles from the water, remove the stems, and chop. Reserve the soaking water.

In a food processor, combine all of the ingredients except for the chipotle water, and blend. As the hummus is blending, slowly add 4 to 5 tablespoons of the reconstituted chipotle water until you achieve the desired consistency.

Ha-cha-cha! Serve immediately or refrigerate until you are ready to dive in.

Guacamole Hummus

By Renee Van de Motter

Renee has a green thumb and an architect's eye, and is one can-do woman. She makes this amazing dip in a thing called a Magic Bullet (an odd little blender)! Here is her twist on guacamole or hummus. Try this on the Hanover Flatbread (page 163) for lunch.

Prep time: 10 minutes • Makes 3 to 4 cups hummus

2 avocados, pitted and peeled

One 15-ounce can chickpeas, drained and rinsed

2 garlic cloves, crushed

Juice of 1 lime

1 tablespoon fresh cilantro

Pinch of salt

Pinch of freshly ground black pepper

Place all of the ingredients in a food processor, high-speed blender, or Magic Bullet and blend until creamy. Season with salt and pepper to taste. Transfer to a bowl. Serve immediately, or chill.

Fresh Anaheim and Edamame Spread

Adapted from Maeve's Daddy by Jane Esselstyn

At a birthday party for Maeve, one of my daughter Sophie's classmates, I spied a curious dip with a bright, fresh consistency and a light-green color. I asked Maeve's daddy what the base was, and when he said "edamame," I immediately asked him to share the recipe. Here is our light, bright, fresh, oil-free version!

Prep time: 10 minutes • Makes 3 cups spread

2 cups edamame, shelled and cooked

½ cup onion, diced

½ cup fresh cilantro

1 garlic clove, crushed

¼ cup fresh lemon juice (about 1 lemon)

1 tablespoon yellow miso

⅓ cup Anaheim pepper, seeded and diced

3 dashes crushed red pepper flakes

1 to 2 tablespoons water, for texture

Pinch of salt

Pinch of freshly ground black pepper

In a food processor, combine all of the ingredients except the water and salt and pepper.

Blend well and taste. Add water, as needed—the texture should be drier and fluffier than hummus. Season with salt and pepper to taste. Serve immediately or cover and refrigerate.

Tip: Serve this with veggies, crackers, or rice cakes, or try on Sunny Day Flatbread (page 163) for lunch.

Nottingham Sandwich Spread

By Jane Esselstyn

Say the word "Nottingham" slowly three times. The sound should be reminiscent of "Not-Eating-Ham." This recipe is by no means a ham spread, but it sure does have the consistency and texture of one! Try this on none other than the Nottingham Flatbread (page 163) for lunch.

Prep time: 10 minutes • Makes 1½ cups spread

1 cup chickpeas, mashed with fork

¼ cup chopped onion

¼ cup chopped pickles or pickle relish

1 celery stalk, finely chopped

1½ tablespoons mustard

1½ tablespoons applesauce

½ teaspoon fresh dill, chopped

Pinch of salt

Pinch of freshly ground black pepper

Mix all of the ingredients in a bowl using a fork—make sure to smash the chickpeas.

Spread on sandwiches, or serve as a dip.

Spinach-Artichoke Dip and Spread

By Kimetha Wurster

Kimetha used to make her patented spinach-artichoke dip every February for a friend's birthday party. True to her new, dairy-free E2 lifestyle, she was determined to make the recipe dairy-free, too. The guests had no idea it wasn't the traditional one and gobbled it up. And there's no baking necessary. Try this on the St. Nick Pizza (page 162) for lunch or dinner.

Prep time: 10 minutes • Makes around 4 cups dip

14 ounces artichoke hearts, packed in water

2 to 6 garlic cloves

9 ounces fresh spinach, or 1½ cups frozen spinach

1 ripe avocado

1 cup nutritional yeast

6 shakes hot sauce

Pinch of freshly ground black pepper (optional)

Pinch of salt (optional)

In a food processor or blender, pulse the drained artichokes with garlic until chopped.

Add the raw spinach (or drained frozen), avocado, and nutritional yeast and pulse until well mixed.

Shake in the hot sauce and season with salt and pepper as desired, and pulse again. Transfer to a bowl and serve with 100 percent whole wheat crackers or veggies, or use as a spread, dip, pizza sauce, or flatbread spread.

Halle's Guacamole

By Halle Foster Moore

My grandmother was Jane Halle, daughter of Sam and Blanche, founders of the Halle Brothers department store in Cleveland, Ohio. In fact, famous actress Halle Berry grew up in Cleveland, and her mother named her after the department store. My mother's sister, Joan, had four children and named her youngest daughter Halle as well. My cousin Halle has grown up to be an amazing woman: doctor, mother, Clevelander. I am proud to offer Halle's Guacamole as the foundation for the numerous fun guac variations you will find below! Try this on the Santa Fe Pizza (page 162) for lunch or dinner.

Prep time: 10 minutes • Serves 4 to 6

2 ripe avocados, peeled and smashed

2 tomatoes, chopped and seeded

1 bunch fresh cilantro, stems removed and finely chopped

Juice of 1 lime

2 garlic cloves, finely chopped

¼ to ½ red onion, finely chopped

¼ to ½ fresh jalapeño pepper (depending on how hot you like it)

Pinch of salt

Pinch of freshly ground black pepper

Prepare all of the ingredients as indicated. Combine in a bowl and serve.

Variations: Following the above recipe, replace one of the avocados with:

Bok-amole: 2 to 3 stalks of bok choy
Edema-mole: 1 cup shelled edamame
Cuke guac: ½ seeded and peeled cucumber
Broc-amole: 1½ cups steamed broccoli
Pea-guacamole: 1½ cups peas
Chick-guac: one 15-ounce can of chickpeas—or see Guacamole Hummus (page 222)
Guaca Ganoouj: 1 roasted and peeled eggplant

Pasta Sauces

Fast and Fresh Marinara Sauce

By Jane Esselstyn

If you want to create a clean marinara sauce, this is the ticket. Making it fresh is ridiculously easy and it tastes much more alive and healthy! Serve over pasta with Spicy Italian Eat Balls (page 152). This recipe is the basis for a plant-strong pizza sauce, as well.

Prep time: 15 minutes • Makes 7 cups sauce

One 28-ounce can crushed tomatoes, no salt added

One 28-ounce can petite diced tomatoes, no salt added

3 tablespoons chopped fresh basil, or 1 tablespoon dried basil

3 tablespoons fresh oregano or 1 tablespoon dried oregano

2 teaspoons fresh thyme or 1½ teaspoons dried thyme

1 teaspoon onion powder

1 teaspoon garlic salt or garlic powder (optional)

¼ teaspoon crushed red pepper flakes

1 to 2 tablespoons pure maple syrup

Combine all of the ingredients in a shallow saucepan over medium-high heat.

Simmer the ingredients together for 3 to 4 minutes.

Decrease the heat to low and simmer for 5 to 10 minutes more until the ingredients are warm throughout. Serve warm.

Tip: Add sliced and cooked mushrooms, zucchini, yellow squash, chopped bell peppers, or any other veggies you love.

Arrabbiata Creamy Cashew Sauce

Adapted from the Las Vegas Whole Foods Market sauce by Jane Esselstyn

Arrabbiata is Italian for "angry style." The heat from the chipotles, smoked paprika, and fire-roasted tomatoes gives this sauce its tantalizing heat! Try this recipe with nonstick-pan-fried baby 'bella mushrooms and whole wheat penne! Or sample it on the Dragon Slayer Pizza (page 162) for lunch or dinner.

Prep time: 10 minutes (plus overnight soaking) • Serves 4 to 6

1 dried chipotle pepper, reconstituted in water overnight

⅓ cup vegetable stock

2 garlic cloves

1 cup raw cashews, soaked overnight

One 14-ounce can petite diced fire-roasted tomatoes with their juices

½ teaspoon smoked paprika

Almond milk, as needed (optional)

Pinch of salt (optional)

Bring the stock to a boil in a sauté pan and add the whole garlic cloves. Cook until the garlic cloves are tender and the stock has almost evaporated. Remove from the heat and set aside.

In a food processor or high-speed blender, pulse the soaked cashews, cooked garlic cloves, chipotle, tomatoes with juices, and paprika until uniformly smooth. Thin out the mixture to a creamy consistency with almond milk, if desired. Taste and add salt, if desired.

Taste, and if needed, add more chipotles or fire-roasted tomatoes to get the desired spiciness.

Transfer the sauce to a saucepan, heat and serve warm over pasta, or place in a container and store in the fridge until ready to use.

Rompin' Red Lentil Pasta Sauce

By Ann Esselstyn

Red lentils are the surprise ingredient that make this pasta sauce hearty and thick. Nutritional yeast adds a creamy feel. I love this sauce on any whole wheat or brown rice pasta or whole wheat orzo. Add a bunch of chopped Kale or greens of choice to the pasta when about four minutes cooking time is left for a luscious one-pot meal. Asparagus goes well with this, as does a big green salad.

Prep time/cook time: 45 minutes • Makes about 8 cups sauce

1 large onion, chopped

3 carrots, chopped

2 celery stalks, chopped

2 tablespoons garlic, chopped

1 teaspoon dried basil

1 teaspoon dried oregano

¼ teaspoon crushed red pepper flakes

One 28-ounce can crushed tomatoes or one 26-ounce box Pomi brand chopped tomatoes

3 cups no-salt-added vegetable broth

½ cup red lentils

One 6-ounce can tomato paste

½ cup chopped fresh parsley

1 cup fresh basil

3 tablespoons nutritional yeast flakes

½ teaspoon freshly ground black pepper

In a large frying pan stir-fry the onion over medium heat for 2 to 3 minutes, then add carrots, celery, and garlic and continue cooking until all of the vegetables soften and begin to brown.

Add the dried basil, oregano, and pepper flakes and stir and cook for 1 minute.

Increase the heat and add the tomatoes, vegetable broth, lentils, and tomato paste and stir to combine.

Bring to a boil, reduce to a simmer, and cook for 30 minutes.

Stir in the parsley, fresh basil, nutritional yeast, and black pepper, and simmer for 3 to 5 minutes more.

Serve warm over pasta and veggies.

Kale Pesto

By Rip and Jane Esselstyn

What a transformation! With the addition of basil to the Kale Butter recipe (from *The Engine 2 Diet*) comes…Kale Pesto. Add this sauce to any pasta for a healthy and novel meal. Try it on the Clevelander Pizza or the Book Group Pizza (page 162) for your next book group, lunch, or dinner.

Prep time: 15 minutes • Makes 4 cups pesto

2 cups Kale, stripped and cooked	Zest of ½ lemon, or more to taste
1½ cups walnuts	Juice of ½ lemon, or more to taste
2 garlic cloves, chopped	1½ cups fresh basil leaves, packed
½ cup water, or more as desired	Salt (optional)

Preheat oven to 350°F.

Place the Kale into a large pot with an inch of water. Cook for about 5 minutes, drain, and set aside.

Toast the walnuts in the oven for 5 to 7 minutes—watching closely so they do not burn.

Place the drained, cooked Kale and toasted walnuts in a food processor and blend. Add the garlic, water, lemon zest, lemon juice, and basil and continue to blend. When the mixture reaches the texture of traditional pesto, taste-test it. If needed, add more lemon, basil, water, or salt, if using, and pulse again.

Serve over pasta, or use as a spread, a dip, or a dressing.

Tip: Add fresh mint to your liking, too!

Cilantro-Lime Pesto

Inspired by Anne Iannerelli

Anne is an amazing cook and massage therapist. While giving massages, she often talks about food and recipes, not realizing the impact her words have on a ravenous belly and very relaxed mind! Anne suggests using Cilantro-Lime Pesto as a topping for sweet potatoes.

Prep time: 5 minutes • Makes about 1 cup pesto

> 2 cups fresh cilantro, packed
> Juice of 1 lime
> 2 garlic cloves, minced
> Crushed red pepper flakes

Combine all of the ingredients in a food processor. Pulse until the mixture is the texture of pesto. Use the pesto as a topping for sweet potato or anything that needs a party on top!

Nutty Ginger Sauce

By Jane Esselstyn

Nutty! Just nutty! And utterly delicious. Top any pasta with this luscious sauce, or make the Dino Kale over Buckwheat Soba Noodles with Nutty Ginger Sauce recipe (page 196).

Prep time: 10 minutes • Serves 6

> ⅓ cup walnuts
> ⅓ cup raw cashews
> ⅓ cup sunflower seeds
> 1 fresh garlic clove, peeled
> 2 teaspoons peeled and grated fresh ginger
> 1 tablespoon low-sodium tamari sauce
>
> 3 to 4 dashes crushed red pepper flakes
> 1 cup water, or more for desired consistency
> 2 teaspoons apricot jam (no-sugar-added) or apricot puree (i.e., dried apricots soaked overnight, then pureed in a food processor)

Blend all of the ingredients in a food processor until smooth.

Tip: Serve over whole wheat pasta, buckwheat soba noodles, Kale, etc.

Kreg's Cashew Cream or Spread

By Kreg Sterns

We suggest making this a bit thick so it's spreadable. This "cream" is a key ingredient in the Pasta Pie recipe (page 198), which is one beauty of a dish. It may also be used on pizzas and flatbread creations!

Prep time: 5 minutes • Makes 2 cups cream

> 1½ cups raw cashews, soaked in water for a few hours or overnight
> 2 to 3 tablespoons nutritional yeast
> 1 fresh garlic clove or ¼ teaspoon garlic powder
> 1 teaspoon sea salt or 1 tablespoon Bragg Liquid Aminos or low-sodium tamari sauce
> ¼ teaspoon freshly ground black pepper

Blend all of the ingredients in a food processor or high-speed blender. Add water, as needed, to reach the desired consistency: thinner for more of a sauce or thicker for more of a spread.

Salads

Lime-Mango Bean Salad

By Ann Esselstyn

This is a family favorite. A version of this is in my father's book, *Prevent and Reverse Heart Disease*. We could eat this every day, and you can be confident everyone will love it.

Prep time: 10 minutes • Serves 4 to 6

> One 15-ounce can cannellini beans, drained and rinsed
> 1 mango, pitted, peeled, and cut into cubes
> 1 avocado, pitted, peeled, and cut into cubes
> ¼ red onion diced, or more as desired
> 1 bunch fresh cilantro (or arugula or spinach)
> Zest and juice of 1 lime

Combine all of the ingredients in a bowl. Be sure to use enough lime; if there is not a lot of juice in your lime, use two.

Serve immediately, or chilled.

Super Salad

Adapted from the Superfood Salad by Whole Foods Market

Do you want your body to feel as fresh as the food you eat? Of course you do! This amazing super salad is inspired by a Whole Foods Market recipe by chef Brad Matthews that I first encountered at the Colorado Springs store. When I give presentations across the country and abroad, I let everyone sample this salad, and people unanimously go Kale krazy for it. All the ingredients come together magically with the accompanying Super-Duper Dressing (page 214) to create one Super-Duper Salad.

Prep time: 20 minutes • Serves 10 or more

> 1 bunch Kale, leaves stripped of spines, spines discarded
> ½ head napa cabbage, finely shredded or finely chopped
> ¼ red onion, thinly sliced
> 3 to 4 carrots, peeled and grated
> ½ cup grape tomatoes, halved
> 1 cup raw edamame, shelled
> 1 cup fresh blueberries
> ½ cup raw, unsalted cashew pieces (optional)
> ¼ cup pumpkin seeds, toasted and unsalted

Finely chop the Kale leaves.

In a large salad bowl, combine all of the ingredients.

Dress the salad with plenty of your favorite dressing—we recommend Super-Duper Dressing (page 214).

Orange-Chipotle Glazed Tofu in Butter Lettuce Nests

By Brad Matthews

This colorful blend of flavors can also be served within spears of romaine lettuce or over a bed of greens—or on its own. As Chef Brad likes to say, "It plates very well." If you are not a fan of chipotle peppers, just don't use them; if you love them, add more.

Prep time: 10 minutes (if using jam) • Cook time: 30 to 40 minutes • Serves 6

- 1 cup fresh orange juice
- 1 tablespoon peeled and grated fresh ginger
- 2 tablespoons no-sugar-added apricot jam or apricot puree (to make apricot puree: soak dried apricots overnight, drain, and then puree in a blender until smooth)
- 2 tablespoons, plus 1 teaspoon low-sodium tamari sauce
- ¼ cup rice vinegar
- 12 ounces firm tofu
- 1 to 2 chipotle peppers, finely chopped
- ½ green bell pepper, diced
- ½ red bell pepper, diced
- 3 scallions, thinly sliced
- ½ bunch fresh cilantro, chopped
- 1 head butter lettuce, leaves detached

Place the orange juice, ginger, apricot jam or puree, tamari, and rice vinegar in a container large enough to hold the tofu. Cut the tofu in 1-inch squares and marinate for at least 2 hours, preferably overnight.

Preheat the oven to 350°F. Line a sheet pan with parchment paper.

Remove the tofu from the marinade and transfer to the lined pan. Bake for 30 to 40 minutes until browned.

Save the marinade and pour into a saucepan. Bring to a boil and reduce by half to create a glaze. Add the chipotles to the glaze and refrigerate until chilled.

Toss the tofu together with the bell peppers, scallions, cilantro, and glaze.

Scoop about ¼ cup of the mixture into the curve of a butter lettuce leaf. Eat with a fork or, better yet, your hands and a big napkin!

Red Quinoa Salad with Black Beans and Corn

By Wendy Solganik of Healthy Girl's Kitchen

Wendy is from one of the best-kept secrets going in Cleveland, Ohio! She is a kindred spirit in the plant-strong world and also has one of the best blogs: *Healthy Girl's Kitchen.* Wendy loves creating delicious and gorgeous food, photographing her wonders, and then blogging about it.

Prep time: 20 minutes • Serves 8

1 cup red quinoa (or 2 cups cooked quinoa)

2 cups vegetable broth

One 15-ounce can black beans, drained and rinsed

2 cups roasted corn

½ large avocado (or 1 small), cut into small pieces

2 cups grape tomatoes, halved

½ cup red onion, finely diced

Juice of 1 orange

Juice of 2 limes

2 tablespoons rice wine vinegar

2 teaspoons pure maple syrup

2 teaspoons Bragg Liquid Aminos or low-sodium tamari sauce

½ bunch fresh cilantro, chopped

Greens of your choice: arugula, mesclun, spring mix, spinach, or romaine

Cook the quinoa as directed on the package, using vegetable broth instead of water, or use precooked quinoa and eliminate the broth.

Meanwhile, place the black beans, corn, avocado, tomatoes, and onion together in a large bowl.

In a blender or food processor, blend together the orange juice, lime juice, vinegar, maple syrup, and tamari to make the dressing.

Add the dressing to the vegetables in the bowl and toss gently. Add the chopped cilantro and toss again.

When the quinoa is cool, place it in a bowl and top with the dressed bean-and-corn salad mixture.

Serve over a bed of greens, if desired, or just as is—YUM!

Tattoo Lentil-Tabbouleh Salad

By John Mercer

John, from the mighty Park Lane Whole Foods Market store, is the first person we know to get a "Forks Over Knives" tattoo on his neck! He is obviously one passionate and enthusiastic plant-strong chef. This recipe comes from his core, and I would expect nothing less from this cross-fit enthusiast. He loves schooling all the Paleo diet lovers he works out with: Paleo vs. Plant-eo. Go, John!

Prep time: 30 minutes • Serves 8 to 10

8 ounces dried green lentils

2½ cups water

1½ tablespoons minced garlic

1 tablespoon Bragg Liquid Aminos

2 cups grape tomatoes, cut in quarters

3 scallions, thinly sliced

½ small red onion, diced

1 cucumber, peeled, seeded, and diced

½ bunch fresh curly parsley, finely chopped (about ¼ cup)

1 bunch mint, finely chopped (about 2 tablespoons)

½ cup fresh lemon juice

¼ teaspoon granulated garlic

Salt

Freshly ground pepper

In a small pot, cover the lentils with 2½ cups water and add garlic and the Bragg Liquid Aminos. Bring to a boil, reduce to a simmer, and cook until the lentils are cooked through, 10 to 15 minutes.

Prep the vegetables, parsley, and mint and toss in a large bowl with the lemon juice and garlic.

Drain the cooked lentils and add to the bowl. Salt and pepper to taste.

Serve cold, plain, or over a bed of baby spinach.

Tip: This salad is best made far enough ahead of time that the flavors have a chance to blend.

Beet and Orange Salad

By Adrienne Hart

This simple recipe tastes complex. Prepare the beets ahead to save time on this dramatic, colorful, phytochemical-filled feast.

Cook time for beets: 20 minutes • Prep time: 15 minutes • Serves 6

4 medium beets, cooked, peeled, and cut into ½-inch chunks

4 navel oranges or blood oranges, segmented

¼ cup chopped fresh mint

¼ cup chopped fresh parsley

¼ cup champagne vinegar

1 shallot or ½ white onion, minced

Zest of 1 lemon

Juice of 1½ lemons (about 6 tablespoons)

Combine the beets, oranges (sectioned by cutting off ends and peeling, then removing the white pith from each section), mint, and parsley in a bowl.

In a separate bowl, add the vinegar, shallot, lemon zest, and lemon juice and whisk to combine.

Toss the salad ingredients with the dressing. Serve chilled.

Thai Slaw

Adapted from Vegan's Daily Companion

The inspiration for this recipe came from a dish served at the Healthy You Network in Tucson, Arizona, and it has changed the way Jane and I view and consume cabbage. Jane says she finds this irresistible and that she could eat Thai Slaw at every meal—every single meal! (She claims her blood is missing some component contained within the ingredients...)

Prep time: 15 minutes • Serves 4 to 6

1¼ cups salsa

¼ cup natural peanut butter

1 tablespoon pure maple syrup

1 tablespoon water

1 teaspoon low-sodium tamari sauce

2 teaspoons peeled and minced fresh ginger

2 to 3 shakes crushed red pepper flakes (optional)

½ head green cabbage, finely shredded

1 red bell pepper, seeded and julienned

1 bunch fresh cilantro, chopped

¼ cup raw peanuts, coarsely chopped

In a saucepan over medium heat, combine the salsa, peanut butter, maple syrup, water, tamari, ginger, and pepper flakes, if using, until uniformly blended into a sauce.

Pour the sauce over the shredded cabbage and toss.

Add the bell pepper, cilantro, and chopped peanuts, and serve.

This is great the next day—it marinates well!

Tip: If cherry tomatoes are your thing, halve them and use instead of the red peppers.

Grape Tomato, Fresh Mint, and Watermelon Ball Salad

By Jane Esselstyn

A hot day begs for this cool meal. Have your kids help make the watermelon balls—if they don't eat them all first!

Prep time: 10 minutes • Serves 4

> 2 cups watermelon balls
> 2 cups grape tomatoes, halved (use a mix of colors if available)
> 4 scallions, thinly sliced
> Fresh mint leaves, finely chopped
> Balsamic glaze, preferably Isola Classic Cream of Balsamic, or similar brand

Combine the watermelon, tomatoes, scallions, and mint in a bowl. Add the balsamic glaze to taste and mix in gently. Serve chilled.

Tip: Serve this over cold soba noodles or rice.

BMT Salad

By Jane Esselstyn

Our family grew up on BLTs (bacon, lettuce, and tomato). And boy did we ever love them. We even used to have "bacon bats," family outings where we'd cook bacon over an open fire and consume BLT after BLT. That was then, this is now. Today we consume BMT after BMT, BMT being this plant-smart basil, mango, and tomato salad.

Prep time: 5 to 10 minutes • Serves 4

> 2 ripe mangos, pitted and cut into cubes
> 4 plum tomatoes, cut into cubes
> 12 large fresh basil leaves, sliced into thin strips
> 2 tablespoons balsamic vinegar
> 2 cups arugula or mâche

Combine the mangos, tomatoes, and basil in a bowl. Sprinkle with balsamic vinegar and stir gently.

Serve on a bed of arugula or mâche.

Grilled Thai Kale Salad

By Brad Matthews

This salad is so gorgeous you may want to just sit and look at it. I suggest decorating it with your favorite dressing, taking a photo, and then diving in. I recommend Sesame Tamari Dressing (from *The Engine 2 Diet*) or Toby's Peanut Dipping Sauce and Dressing (page 217).

Prep time: 15 minutes • Serves 8

  1 bunch Kale, leaves stripped of spines, spines discarded
  1 red onion, chopped
  ½ fresh pineapple, peeled, cored, and cut into cubes
  ½ jalapeño pepper, seeded and chopped
  1 cup sugar snap peas
  1 cup cherry tomatoes

Finely chop the Kale leaves. Place the Kale in a large bowl.

On a grill, or in a hot pan, grill the red onion, pineapple, jalapeño, sugar snap peas, and cherry tomatoes until the colors are bright and the vegetables are a little charred and caramelized.

In a large bowl, combine the chopped Kale and cooked vegetables.

Toss this stunning salad with your favorite plant-strong dressing and enjoy.

Kale Ceviche Salad

By Rip Esselstyn

I've always thought of Kale as lettuce with an attitude, but I recently read a reference to Kale as "angry lettuce." This cracks me up! Kale is superior to all other foods on the planet when it comes to its micronutrient content, so I'm always looking for delicious ways to incorporate it in my diet. Massaging this salad drives the lemon juice and salt into the cell membrane of the Kale and lightly "cooks" it, making it much more tame and less "angry."

Prep time: 10 minutes • Serves 6 to 8

1 bunch Kale, leaves stripped of spines, spines discarded

1 large (or 2 small) avocados, peeled and chopped

Juice of ½ lemon

¼ to ½ teaspoon salt (optional)

½ teaspoon crushed red pepper flakes

½ red bell pepper, seeded and finely chopped

1 small carrot, grated

½ purple onion, diced

1½ to 2 cups mandarin orange segments (about 3 oranges)

Throw the stripped and chopped Kale leaves in a large bowl with avocado, lemon juice, salt, if using, and red pepper flakes.

Mash and massage the avocado into the Kale with your hands until the avocado is spread evenly—like a dressing—throughout the Kale.

Stir in the bell pepper, carrot, purple onion, and mandarin oranges.

If you can, let the salad sit for 30 minutes before serving—if not, dive in!

Tip: If you don't like avocado, hummus works just as well!

Grilled Romaine Salad

By Phyllis Taft

The street in Cleveland where we grew up holds an annual Labor Day picnic. The whole community shares two grills. Everyone is nice enough to let the Esselstyn family cook our veggie burgers first, then offer grill space to the next family. One time, expecting beef hot dogs, turkey burgers, or other flesh to arrive next, Jane called out the famous line from *Monty Python and the Holy Grail*: "Bring out your dead!" But instead of meat, one of our neighbors approached with a beautiful armful of romaine lettuce. Entranced, we hung around and watched as she grilled the long, bright, quartered heads, then added orange slices, pepper, and salt. Before she poured on any oil or feta, Jane and I grabbed the leaves and ran off with a winner of a new recipe!

Prep time: 10 minutes • Serves 4

1 head romaine, cut lengthwise into quarters

1 orange, segmented (by cutting off ends, peeling, and then removing white pith from each section)

Salt (optional)

Freshly ground black pepper (optional)

Balsamic glaze, preferably Isola Classic Cream of Balsamic, or similar brand

Place the quartered romaine sections on an open preheated grill. Flip the sections as you grill so that the leaves cook on all sides. The sections should be warmed through and crisp.

Transfer the grilled romaine leaves into a large bowl, toss with the juicy orange segments, any juice from the orange, and a pinch of salt and pepper, if desired, then drizzle with the balsamic glaze.

Tip: This recipe works in the oven under the broiler, too!

Salsas

Down Under Cranberry Salsa

Inspired by the Wright family recipe

Whenever Aussie Leanne Wright serves this at her Christmas party, she is inevitably mobbed for the recipe. Jane happened to be part of such a mob, secured the famed recipe, and tweaked a few things. Now here it is: a new family favorite, especially around the holidays.

Prep time: 15 minutes • Makes 2½ to 3 cups salsa

> One 12-ounce package fresh cranberries
> Juice of 1½ limes
> ½ cup pure maple syrup
> 3 to 4 scallions, thinly sliced
> ½ large jalapeño pepper, seeded and chopped
> 2 cups fresh cilantro, measured whole, without stems, not chopped

Put all of the ingredients in a food processor, and run only until coarsely chopped. Chill and serve with toasted whole wheat pita, on top of rice and beans, or with anything that needs zip.

Tip: Blending the mixture longer turns this salsa into more of a relish, which can be delish!

Grape-Mango Salsa

By Fred Wenz

Fred is a creative and clever engineer who's also known for his amazing recipes. Here is a smashing salsa with lots of room for artistic license. It is so colorful, bountiful, and plentiful it could double as a side dish!

Prep time: 30 minutes • Makes 5 cups salsa

> 6 plum or other meaty tomatoes, sliced into chunks
> 1 seedless orange, peeled and sliced into chunks
> 1 mango, peeled, pitted, and sliced into chunks
> 1 garlic clove, finely chopped
> 3 scallions, diced (or ¼ red onion, diced)
> 1 bunch seedless red grapes, halved
> Juice of 1 lime
> ½ cup cilantro, stems removed and chopped
> Freshly ground black pepper
> Salt
> ½ jalapeño pepper, seeded and minced (optional)

Prep all of the ingredients for the salsa. Combine in a bowl and mix gently to avoid damaging the fruit. Add the cilantro, pepper and salt to taste, and minced jalapeño pepper, if desired. Mix and serve.

Quick Salsa Fresca

By Jane Esselstyn

There are times of the year when the tomatoes are so fresh and the mangos so perfect, only a fresh salsa will do. This salsa is quick, fresh, and alive. It will brighten up your meal and your day!

Prep time: 10 minutes • Makes 3 to 4 cups salsa

2 cups cherry tomatoes, halved
2 champagne mangos, peeled, pitted, and cut into cubes
6 scallions (more or less, as you prefer), thinly sliced
Zest and juice of 1 lime

Combine the tomatoes, mangos, and scallions in a bowl. Add the zest and juice of the lime. Mix and serve.

Tip: In place of mangos, try watermelon balls. Also try adding avocado!

Apple-Celery Salsa

By Debbie Kastner

This recipe was originally meant to be a topping for the Red Lentil Mulligatawny (page 250). Its flavor is unique and so crisp we recommend using it for everything else you can think of, from a topping for a burger or burrito to a salad dressing to a dessert topping.

Prep time: 10 minutes • Makes 1+ cups salsa

⅔ cup finely chopped Granny Smith apples
¼ cup finely chopped celery
1 tablespoon chopped fresh cilantro
1 tablespoon fresh lime juice
¼ cup cherry tomatoes, halved

Combine all of the ingredients in a bowl. Mix and serve.

Soups

Walk on Top Thick Lentil-Miso Soup with Mushrooms, Collards, and Kale

By Jane Esselstyn

My mom likes soup she can walk on! In other words, she prefers it thick, and so do all Esselstyns! This hearty lentil soup with darn near the whole garden chopped, diced, and minced up within will keep you stepping high.

Prep time: 15 minutes • Cook time: 20 minutes • Serves 8 to 10

One 15-ounce can lentils, or 1 cup dry lentils
1 onion, chopped
½ cup sliced carrots
½ cup sliced celery
One 8-ounce package mushrooms, sliced
3 garlic cloves, minced
4 to 6 cups vegetable stock
1 tomato, diced
1 sweet potato, peeled and cut into cubes
1 tablespoon paprika
1 tablespoon onion powder
1 teaspoon garlic salt
1 teaspoon freshly ground black pepper
2 tablespoons miso
3 collard green leaves, stripped of spines and chopped
4 to 6 Kale leaves, stripped of spines and chopped
½ bunch fresh parsley, chopped, for garnish

If you are starting with dry lentils, begin recipe here; if you are using cooked lentils, go to the next paragraph. Add the lentils and 2½ cups of water to a large pot and bring to a boil. Decrease the heat and simmer 10 to 15 minutes until the lentils are cooked through.

In a large soup pot, sauté the onions, carrots, celery, mushrooms, and garlic. Add the stock, cooked lentils, tomato, sweet potato, paprika, onion powder, garlic salt, and pepper and simmer for 15 minutes. Ladle ½ cup of the warm broth from the soup pot into a small bowl, add the miso, and stir until dissolved. Add the dissolved miso to the soup pot. Add the collard greens and Kale leaves and simmer until the greens are soft and deep green in color. Garnish with parsley and serve.

Tortilla Soup with Crispy Sticks

Inspired by Rachel Safran from the Las Vegas Whole Foods Market store

This is a delicious twist on traditional Tortilla Soup. Some like their soup thicker and others thinner. Whatever your preference, prepare this classic to your liking. But no matter what, you will love the crispy strips.

Prep time: 15 minutes • Cook time: 15 minutes • Serves 6 to 8

6 to 8 corn tortillas

3 to 4 cups vegetable broth

1 yellow onion, diced

½ cup diced red bell pepper

3 garlic cloves, minced

One 15-ounce can fire-roasted chopped tomatoes

One 15-ounce can fire-roasted crushed tomatoes

One 15-ounce can black beans, drained and rinsed

1 cup frozen corn kernels, thawed

8 ounces canned whole green chilies, chopped

2 tablespoons ground cumin

½ cup diced avocado (about 1 small avocado)

Preheat the oven to 400°F.

Cut the corn tortillas into ¼- to ½-inch-wide strips and place on a baking sheet. Bake for 3 to 5 minutes until crispy. Remove from the oven and set aside.

Place ½ cup of broth in a medium saucepan and add the onion, bell pepper, and garlic. Cook for 5 minutes over low heat, stirring occasionally. Add the remaining 2½ to 3½ cups broth (depending on how thick you like your soup) and both kinds of canned tomatoes, then bring to a boil. Add the beans, corn, chilies, and cumin and cook over medium heat for 15 minutes. Using an immersion blender, blend very briefly, or mash slightly; this will thicken the soup a bit. Add the avocado, stir to incorporate, and cook 2 to 3 minutes more.

Serve with the crispy tortilla strips on top.

Tip: To make this dish spicier, add ¼ teaspoon of crushed red pepper flakes, or a reconstituted chipotle pepper for a smoky kick!

Spicy African Peanut Perfection

By Debbie Kastner

Here is another Happy Healthy Librarian recipe! Debbie "enlightened" this recipe from a soup posted on the *Peas and Thank You* blog with a fantastic invention: homemade "Faux Coconut Milk"! It is made by mixing unsweetened soy or almond or oat milk with coconut extract! It is an amazingly healthy replacement for real coconut milk.

Prep time/cook time: 70 minutes • Serves 6

One 15-ounce can chickpeas, drained and rinsed

1 large sweet potato, peeled and cut into cubes (3 to 4 cups)

1½ teaspoons curry powder

1 teaspoon garam masala

1 teaspoon ground cumin

¼ teaspoon ground cinnamon

1 tablespoon peeled and minced fresh ginger

3 garlic cloves, minced

1½ tablespoons pure maple syrup

One 14-ounce can petite diced tomatoes

One 4-ounce can whole green chilies, chopped

1½ cups unsweetened soy, or almond, or oat milk

1 teaspoon coconut extract

2 cups low-sodium vegetable broth

2 tablespoons natural peanut butter

½ cup dried red lentils, rinsed

Cooked brown rice, for serving (optional)

Chopped fresh cilantro, for garnish

¼ cup raw peanuts, chopped, for garnish (optional)

In a large soup pot, combine all of the ingredients. Bring to a boil, lower to a simmer, and cook for 1 hour until the lentils turn to mush, and the sweet potatoes are "just right"—soft, but not mushy.

Serve on its own or over cooked brown rice, if desired, garnished with the chopped cilantro and chopped peanuts.

Butternut Barley Soup

Inspired by Rachel Safran at the Las Vegas Whole Foods store

This combination of butternut and barley goes together as well as their fun B&B alliteration suggests. The creamy, smooth, substantial squash base of this soup balances well with the chewy, satisfying barley. This soup is a winner.

Prep time/cook time: 75 minutes • Makes about 7 cups soup

1 cup hulled barley

8 cups vegetable stock

3 whole garlic cloves

1 yellow onion, diced

1 tablespoon peeled and minced fresh ginger

3 pounds butternut squash, peeled, seeded, and diced

1 red bell pepper, seeded and diced

2 tablespoons fresh thyme leaves

In a small pot, combine 1 cup barley with 2 cups of the stock. Cover and bring to a boil. Reduce to a simmer and cook for 15 minutes.

Meanwhile, in a separate small pot, bring ½ cup of the stock to a boil. Add the whole garlic cloves and simmer for 12 to 15 minutes until the garlic is fork-tender. Carefully remove the garlic and set aside.

In a soup pot over medium-high heat, sweat the onion in ½ cup of the stock. Once the onion is soft and translucent, add the fresh ginger and sauté for 5 minutes. Add the diced butternut squash and bell pepper and cover with the remaining 5 cups stock. Simmer for 35 to 40 minutes until the squash is fork-tender.

Chop the garlic cloves and add to the soup along with the thyme. Remove half of the soup, transfer to a food processor, and blend. Blend all of the soup, if you want it completely smooth. Or if you have a handheld immersion blender, use it to blend the soup to your liking.

Return the blended portion of the soup to the pot and add the cooked barley. Continue cooking for 20 to 25 minutes more. Serve warm.

Tip: Try this soup with Better-milk Biscuits (page 155).

Renee's Gazpacho

By Renee Van de Motter

Jane's friend Renee is a scientist, math teacher, and mom. Last spring when we challenged her to make gazpacho without oil, she didn't hesitate for a moment. She said, "Okay, a little sourdough bread should do the trick, and spring tomatoes may not be as acidic as late-summer tomatoes, so you may not need as much bread." Say what?!!

Prep time: 15 minutes • Serves 4 to 6

6 tomatoes, cut into cubes

1 medium cucumber, peeled, seeded, and cut into cubes

2 celery stalks, sliced

½ red bell pepper, seeded and diced

½ onion, chopped

2 garlic cloves, peeled and crushed

2 to 3 tablespoons red wine vinegar

3 slices sourdough bread, cubed and crusts removed

Pinch of salt

Pinch of freshly ground black pepper

2 tomatoes, chopped (to be added into puree)

1 celery stalk, chopped (to be added into puree)

½ green bell pepper, seeded and chopped (to be added into puree)

¼ cucumber, peeled, seeded, and chopped (to be added into puree)

Chopped fresh parsley or cilantro, for garnish

Place the tomato, cucumber, celery, red bell pepper, onion, garlic, vinegar, and sourdough bread in a food processor or high-speed blender and puree until the ingredients are well blended. Season with salt and pepper to taste.

Mix in chopped tomatoes, celery, green bell pepper, and cucumber by hand.

Chill and serve garnished with chopped parsley or cilantro.

Red Lentil Mulligatawny Topped with Apple-Celery Salsa

By The Healthy Librarian and The Soup Peddler

The Soup Peddler in Austin, Texas, is a local icon because when he started his business more than twenty years ago, he delivered all of his soup on the back of his bike. Today, he has a fleet of little trucks! One of his stellar soups is the mulligatawny. The Healthy Librarian has this great version of it, made with her famous Faux Coconut Milk and a stunning Apple-Celery Salsa.

Prep time: 20 minutes • Cook time: 20 minutes • Serves 4 to 5

3½ cups fat-free, low-sodium vegetable broth	1 teaspoon peeled and grated fresh ginger
1 cup small, dried red lentils	½ teaspoon ground cumin
1 cup chopped onion	⅛ teaspoon ground turmeric
1 carrot, chopped	¼ teaspoon ground coriander
1 celery stalk, chopped	¼ teaspoon cayenne pepper
½ cup cauliflower, chopped	⅛ teaspoon ground cinnamon
1½ cups unsweetened soy, almond, or oat milk	1 tablespoon fresh lime juice
1 teaspoon coconut extract	½ teaspoon salt (optional)
3 tablespoons tomato paste	Apple-Celery Salsa (page 244), chilled, for garnish

In a soup pot, combine the broth, lentils, onions, carrot, celery, and cauliflower. Bring to a boil over a medium heat. Cover, reduce to a simmer, and cook 15 minutes, or until the lentils are tender. Set aside to cool for 15 minutes.

Meanwhile, stir together the unsweetened non-dairy milk and the coconut extract. Set aside.

Pour half of the mixture in the pot into a high-speed blender or food processor and blend until smooth. Return to the pot with the rest of the mixture. Alternatively, blend briefly using an immersion blender.

Add the coconut mixture, tomato paste, ginger, cumin, turmeric, coriander, cayenne to taste, and cinnamon to a blender. Blend until smooth. Pour this mixture into the soup pot, cover, and simmer over low heat for 10 minutes, or until heated through.

Remove the pot from the heat and stir in the lime juice. Season with salt to taste, if using. Ladle the soup into bowls and top with ¼ cup of the Apple-Celery Salsa.

Thai Carrot Soup

By Andrew Casesse

Andrew's story is like that of many other Americans: He was diagnosed as prediabetic, overweight, and hypertensive. But after attending a weeklong Engine 2 retreat and committing to the plant-strong lifestyle for six months, Andrew now fits none of the above descriptors and is training for a sprint triathlon! His success and this recipe are great "carrots" to dangle in front of you!

Prep time/cook time: 40 minutes • Makes 7 cups soup

- 2 pounds carrots, peeled and chopped
- 1 tablespoon peeled and minced fresh ginger
- 1 onion, chopped
- 1 tablespoon minced garlic
- ¼ cup fresh chopped cilantro, plus a few extra sprigs for garnish
- 32 ounces low-sodium vegetable broth
- 2 to 3 tablespoons low-sodium tamari sauce
- 2 to 3 tablespoons smooth peanut butter
- 1 to 2 cups cooked brown rice
- A sprinkling of crushed red pepper flakes
- ½ cup raw peanuts, crushed

Put the carrots, ginger, onion, garlic, cilantro, and vegetable broth in a soup pot, cover, and simmer for 30 minutes, or until the carrots are soft.

Using an immersion blender or a food processor, blend until smooth. Return the blended mixture to the pot and add the tamari, peanut butter, and cooked rice.

Add red pepper flakes to taste and simmer until heated through.

Serve the soup warm, garnished with the cilantro and a dusting of crushed peanuts.

Sweet Holy Deliciousness

By Ann Esselstyn

The idea for this came from the *Happy Herbivore*'s Sweet Potato Dal recipe, which she calls "Dal-icious"! My mom turned this dal into soup and was more generous with the garam masala than the amount used in the original. Although conventional curry would work, garam masala is a key spice here. Get it—it's worth hunting down in the spice aisle and is a must-have in the kitchen. This soup is delicious for lunch or dinner by itself, or over cooked brown rice or quinoa.

Prep time/cook time: 45 to 60 minutes • Serves 6

2 large onions, chopped

6 large garlic cloves, chopped

2 pinches crushed red pepper flakes

½ teaspoon ground turmeric

1 teaspoon garam masala

6 cups vegetable broth

1 cup dried red lentils

2 large sweet potatoes, peeled and cut into cubes

2 bunches Kale or greens of choice, stripped of spines, spines discarded, and cut into bite-size pieces

Freshly ground black pepper

In a soup pot, stir-fry the onions and garlic for a few minutes until the onions are limp. Add the pepper flakes, turmeric, and garam masala and stir to coat the onions and garlic. Add the vegetable broth and lentils and bring to a boil. Decrease the heat to low, cover, and simmer for about 5 minutes. Add the sweet potatoes, return to a boil, reduce the heat to low, and simmer until the lentils are fully cooked and the sweet potatoes are tender, 5 to 10 minutes. Add the Kale and cook 5 minutes more, or until the Kale is soft. Season with black pepper to taste.

Serve on its own or over a mound of cooked whole grains.

Tip: Add hot sauce for an added kick!

Desserts and Chocolates

Cowgirl Biscotti

By Jane Esselstyn

Yippee-ki-yay! Whip these up and hit the trail, y'all. If you have an aerated pan, it saves one cycle of baking: Both sides of the treat will be done in just fifteen minutes. Ye haw!

Prep time: 5 minutes • Cooling time: 10 minutes • Cook time: 55 minutes

Makes 16 to 20 biscotti

⅔ cup raw cashews or walnuts
2 tablespoons water
½ cup pure maple syrup
1 tablespoon vanilla extract
1½ cups white whole wheat flour
¼ cup old-fashioned rolled oats

½ teaspoon baking soda
⅓ cup of mix-ins: any combination of raisins and pecans, dried cranberries and pistachios, or almonds and non-dairy chocolate chips—or any mix you dream up!

Preheat the oven to 350°F. Line a baking sheet with parchment paper.

In a food processor, blend the cashews and water until the mixture is lumpy. Add the maple syrup and vanilla and blend until uniformly mixed. Pulse in the flour, oats, and baking soda with as few rotations of the blade as possible; this keeps the flour from toughening up. Add your choice of mix-ins and blend once or twice more.

Remove the biscotti dough from the processor and form it into a log, on the parchment-lined pan. Place the log in the oven and bake for 25 minutes.

Remove the log from the oven and set aside to cool. Decrease the oven temperature to 300°F.

When the biscotti log is cool enough to handle, slice with a serrated knife into ¼- to ½-inch slices. Place the slices flat on the same baking pan. Bake for 10 minutes, flip, and bake again for 10 more minutes until both sides are slightly browned.

Cool and serve when phenomenally crisp!

Yonanas!

By Yonanas

Jane told me about this machine, an ice cream maker, and it has changed the way Kole, Sophie, Jill, and I make our E2 "ice cream." It makes crazy smooth soft serve! The foundation is typically frozen bananas, and then you add whatever you want to flavor it—frozen peaches, cherries, blueberries, or even dark chocolate! You can buy a Yonanas machine at Amazon.com for about $49.

Prep time: 2 minutes • Serves 1 to 2

> 2 frozen bananas
> Any other frozen fruit you desire (see list above)

Place the ingredients into your Yonanas machine and run according to the manufacturer's directions.

Get your spoon ready!

Sorbetto Verde

By Char Nolan

Engine 2 nabbed this recipe from Philly's plant-strong Char Nolan. Char attended one of the Engine 2 Immersion programs and commented that she wanted people to see her not as a "fat older female" but rather as a "silver-haired maiden." Three years later, she radiates a beauty and integrity that qualifies her not only as a silver-haired maiden but as a goddess!

Prep time: 3 minutes • Makes 4 cups sorbetto

> 2 cups seedless green grapes
> 2 cups fresh spinach leaves
> ¼ lime, with rind on
> 1 teaspoon pure maple syrup
> 2 cups ice

Place the ingredients in a food processor or high-speed blender in the order listed. The grapes need to be processed first so that they are near the blade since they will become your liquid.

Turn the blender on high. You may need to use a rubber spatula occasionally to scrape any ingredients stuck to the sides. Continue blending the remaining ingredients. You will end up with a solid mass of Sorbetto Verde.

Serve immediately or freeze until ready to serve.

Mango-Cherry "Ice Cream"

By Natala Constantine

Natala Constantine is one of my all-time favorite people in the world. She's got more passion, guts, and charisma than almost anyone I know, and she is constantly reinventing herself. I met Natala more than four years ago and have watched her health skyrocket and her weight plummet. Natala used to be a type 2 diabetic who took fourteen medications daily and weighed more than 420 pounds. Today, she is on zero medications, has completely reversed her diabetes, and has lost more than 200 pounds. She is part of the Engine 2 team and runs our social media campaign. Her wonderful recipe below combines frozen fruit and non-dairy milk into a treat that looks remarkably like ice cream!

Prep time: 5 minutes • Serves 3 to 4

1 cup unsweetened almond, oat, or soy milk
2 pitted dates
1 teaspoon vanilla extract
15 frozen mango chunks (1½ to 2 cups)
20 frozen dark sweet cherries

Combine the non-dairy milk, vanilla, and pitted dates in a food processor and blend. Add the mango chunks and blend again. Add the cherries and blend once more until creamy. Serve immediately.

Lightly Gingered Fruit, Fruit, Fruit Salad

By Ben Baker

A fresh spin on the fruit salad in *The Engine 2 Diet*, this dessert has freshly grated ginger on top. Get yourself a Microplane grater and have fun!

Prep time: 20 minutes • Makes 6 cups salad

1 cup cubed cantaloupe
1 cup cubed pineapple
1 cup sliced strawberries
3 kiwis, peeled and sliced
1 cup seedless grapes
1 cup fresh or frozen raspberries
1 cup fresh orange juice
1 piece peeled fresh ginger

In a large bowl, combine all of the fruit. Pour the orange juice over the fruit and toss gently to combine. Using a Microplane or other fine grater, grate the fresh ginger over the fruit and toss again.

Serve immediately, or refrigerate until it is time to hit the potluck!

Variation: If you are not a fan of ginger, try adding a chiffonade (ribbons) of fresh mint leaf. If you like it, why not both?

Mango Mango

By the Sexy Caribbean Cooking Student

Jane was teaching a cooking class when a beautiful woman with a Caribbean accent told her, "We need more Caribbean foods in this way of eating." Jane replied, "Absolutely! But there is not a Caribbean bone in my body, so you will have to help me." Well, right after the class the woman picked up a mango from the demo table and started squeezing and squeezing it, gently massaging and mashing it with her thumbs. Jane asked, "What is this Caribbean trick?" The woman smiled and said, "Now you make a hole with your teeth, and suck out all the juice and pulp—so sexy!" (Jane is sensitive to mango skin, so she used a straw. Not so sexy!)

Prep time: 5 minutes • Serves 1

    1 ripe, soft mango

Gently press the mango skin, without puncturing it, until it feels juicy from top to bottom and side to side all around the pit. Tear a little hole with your teeth, or insert a straw, and suck out all the goodness.

Apple-Cardamom Flapjack Crumble

By Torrie McMillian

Torrie McMillian runs the Center for Sustainability at Hathaway Brown School near Cleveland and shares an office with my sister Jane. She has a garden nearly as big as her home and holds potlucks that overflow with wholesome bounty. This apple crumble will make you crumble with delight. The cardamom pods add flavor, yet they are not intended to be eaten.

Whoever gets a cardamom pod is a lucky duck and gets to make a wish as he or she places it back on the plate. Serve this with a dollop of Sweet Zu-creamy Cashew Sauce (page 259).

Prep time: 10 minutes • Cook time: 40 minutes • Makes one 9-inch pie

APPLE-CARDAMOM FILLING

4 apples of different types such as Macintosh, Granny Smith, Braeburn, Delicious, Honey Crisp, etc., peeled and diced

6 to 8 cardamom pods

¼ tablespoon coriander seeds

½ teaspoon ground cinnamon

2 teaspoons pure maple syrup

Juice of 1 lime

FLAPJACK CRUMBLE

⅔ cup nuts, your choice

2 tablespoons water

¼ cup pure maple syrup

¼ teaspoon ground cinnamon

½ teaspoon vanilla extract

1⅓ cups old-fashioned rolled oats

Preheat the oven to 375°F. Line a sheet pan with parchment paper.

To make the filling: Place the apples in a bowl. Add the cardamom pods, coriander seeds, cinnamon, maple syrup, and lime juice. Mix until the apples are uniformly coated. Pour the apple mixture into a pie plate or baking dish and cover with a lid or a piece of aluminum foil. Bake for 35 minutes, or until the apples are soft but not mushy.

While the apples are baking, make the crumble: Place the nuts and water in a blender or food processor and blend until the mixture forms a lump. Add the syrup, cinnamon, and vanilla and blend until uniformly mixed. Add the oats and gently pulse 3 or 4 times, or just hand mix.

Remove the crumble from the blender or processor and spread it all over the lined sheet pan, like spilled granola. Bake for about 15 minutes, or until browned and fragrant. Set aside.

Remove the apple-cardamom filling from the oven. Top the filling with the crumble mixture.

Serve warm with a dollop of Sweet Zu-creamy Cashew Sauce (recipe follows).

Sweet Zu-creamy Cashew Sauce

By Rachel Laing, inspired by Ashley

One of our Engine 2 friends, Rachel, discovered this recipe after attending a raw-food class at a friend's house. Ashley, a raw-food chef from San Francisco, was using peeled zucchini in her hummus recipes to increase the creaminess without adding fat or oil. Rachel now chucks peeled zucchini (or unpeeled, for a beautiful green color) into salad dressings and other recipes to invite a creamy-smooth texture. What a great trick!

Prep time: 5 minutes (plus 1 hour to soak cashews) • Makes about 1½ cups sauce

- ¾ cup raw cashews, soaked for at least 1 hour in water
- 1 medium zucchini, well peeled with no green showing, sliced into chunks
- 2 to 3 tablespoons pure maple syrup
- 1 teaspoon vanilla extract
- ½ to 1 cup unsweetened almond milk

Rinse and drain the cashews. Place the cashews in a food processor or high-speed blender with the remaining ingredients, adding the almond milk, as needed, for the desired consistency, depending on how thick you want the sauce.

A thick sauce is great for layering in a parfait glass with fruit, and a thinner sauce is perfect poured over fruit salad or cake.

Tip: For a lemony-tasting sauce, add a bit of lemon zest and a squeeze of fresh lemon juice. Or add less almond milk for frosting!

Banana-Oatmeal Peanut Butter Cookies

Inspired by Lux Hippie Blog

I love bananas, I love oats, and I love peanut butter. So does Jane's thirteen-year-old daughter, Crile, who ate seven of these in one sitting. Teenage approval: That says a lot about how good these cookies are.

Prep time: 10 minutes • Cook time: 15 minutes • Makes about 15 cookies

3 ripe bananas, mashed	2 cups old-fashioned rolled oats
1 tablespoon vanilla extract	½ cup whole wheat flour
¾ cup natural chunky peanut butter	1 teaspoon baking powder
3 tablespoons pure maple syrup	½ cup non-dairy chocolate chips or raisins

Preheat the oven to 350°F. Line a baking sheet with parchment paper.

In a large bowl, mix the bananas, vanilla, peanut butter, and maple syrup until they are a creamy consistency.

In a separate bowl, combine the oats, flour, and baking powder.

Add the dry ingredients to the wet ingredients and stir until they are well combined; the batter should be slightly sticky. Fold in the chocolate chips or raisins.

Place rounded, heaping tablespoon-size balls of the batter onto the lined baking sheet. Bake for 15 to 18 minutes.

Gobble these up while they are still warm.

CAUTION! CHOCOLATE AHEAD!

Adonis Cake

By Betty Speer and Adonis

This is a chocolate cake for the gods—moist and chocolatey with dreamy, creamy Adonis Frosting (see page 261 for recipe). Jill made this cake for my forty-ninth birthday party and it was a smash! The recipe comes from Jill's aunt Betty and her wonderful eight-year-old grandson, Adonis.

Prep time: 10 minutes • Cook time: 30 minutes • Makes one 9 × 9-inch cake

1½ cups whole wheat flour	6 tablespoons unsweetened applesauce
3 tablespoons unsweetened cocoa powder	1 tablespoon white vinegar
1 teaspoon baking soda	1 teaspoon vanilla extract
⅔ cup pure maple syrup	¾ cup cold water

Preheat the oven to 350°F. Set out a 9 x 9-inch nonstick cake pan.

In a mixing bowl, combine the flour, cocoa, and baking soda and mix well. Add the maple syrup, applesauce, vinegar, vanilla, and water and mix well to combine.

Pour the batter into the prepared cake pan. Bake for 30 minutes.

While the cake is cooking, make the Adonis Frosting (recipe follows).

When the cake is done, remove it from the oven and set aside to cool. When cooled, frost with Adonis Frosting or Zu-creamy Cashew Sauce (page 259).

Tip: If you want a two-layer cake, then just double the recipe—and the frosting recipe below as well. Then frost in between and all over both layers!

Adonis Frosting

By Betty Speer

Chocolate frosting of the gods!

Prep time: 5 minutes • Makes about 2 cups frosting; enough for one Adonis Cake, plus a few taste-tests

> One 12-ounce package silken tofu
> ¾ cup dairy-free, semisweet chocolate chips, melted
> 1 tablespoon vanilla extract

Place the silken tofu in a food processor. Add the melted chocolate chips to the food processor and blend.

Add the vanilla and blend until chocolatey and creamy. Taste at this stage; if using grain-sweetened chips, you may want to add a bit of pure maple syrup—or not! Trust your own taste.

Use immediately or refrigerate until ready to use.

Tip: This recipe can be used as a pudding as well. After preparing it, pour it into glasses, layer with sliced fruit, and refrigerate until ready to serve.

Date-Nut Chocolate Pie

Inspired by Chef A.J. and Ben Baker

This recipe was initially inspired by the Fundue recipe of Los Angeles's own plant-strong dessert chef, Abbie Jay (A.J.). She prepared Fundue at the Travassa resort where Ben Baker is head chef. Ben pulled out all the stops and helped us create a seven-day meal plan for plant-sensational meals that met the Engine 2 diet criteria. For dessert one night, Ben whipped up this amazing Date-Nut Chocolate Pie using a crust in the Engine 2 book and Chef A.J.'s Fundue filling. We also recommend trying this pie with a crisp Flapjack Crumble crust (page 258). Jane claims this recipe saved her from the grasp of an almond M&M addiction. This pie is that freaky good!

Prep time: 20 minutes (plus overnight soaking for dates) • Cook time: 25 minutes (only if using Flapjack Crumble crust) • Freeze time: 8 hours to overnight • Makes one 9-inch pie and some extra filling

CHOCOLATE FILLING

    10 ounces pitted dates (about 16 large Medjool dates)
    2 cups unsweetened almond milk
    8 ounces almond butter or peanut butter
    1 tablespoon vanilla extract
    ⅓ to ½ cup unsweetened cocoa powder

DATE-NUT CRUST

    1 cup dates, pitted
    ⅓ cup raw walnuts
    ⅓ cup raw cashews
    ⅓ cup raw almonds
    1 teaspoon vanilla extract

GARNISH

    Fresh fruit, for topping

CHOCOLATE FILLING

Two nights before, start to make the filling: Place the dates in a container and pour almond milk over them. Seal the container and soak the dates in the fridge overnight.

The next day continue to make the filling by placing the soaked dates and almond milk in a food processor. Make sure there are no pits in the dates or your food processor will buck, splatter, and thump.

Blend the soaked dates and almond milk until well combined and creamy. Add the almond butter (or peanut butter) and vanilla to the food processor and blend again. If needed, add more almond milk for a thick but creamy consistency. Add the cocoa powder and blend well—it is just luscious at this stage. Set aside while you make the crust.

DATE-NUT CRUST

To make the Date-Nut Crust: Blend the dates, walnuts, cashews, almonds, and vanilla in a food processor until one big clump forms. Press the date-nut clump into a pie pan and fill with chocolate filling.

FLAPJACK CRUMBLE CRUST

To make the Flapjack Crumble crust: Follow the directions for making Flapjack Crumble on page 258, but shape the ingredients in the pie pan and bake as directed on page 258.

Now pour the Chocolate Filling into the Date-Nut Crust or Flapjack Crumble crust–lined pie pan. Cover the pie and freeze overnight or for at least 8 hours before serving so it hardens.

Remove the pie from the freezer in time for it to thaw enough to cut. Slice into wedges and serve. Add fresh fruit on top just before serving.

Variation: Pour any extra chocolate filling into a brownie pan, freeze, then serve cut into squares, rolled into truffle-like balls, or shaved into twirls with toasted and crushed almonds or walnuts on top!

Chocomole

By Anne Stevenson

Anne Stevenson (page 145) brought down the house when she brought this thick, creamy, chocolatey, fall-of-the-Roman-Empire, decadent dessert to my forty-sixth birthday party. We all did cartwheels it was so good.

Prep time: 5 minutes • Makes 1 cup chocomole

1 ripe avocado, pitted and peeled
⅓ cup pure maple syrup
¼ cup unsweetened cocoa powder
1 teaspoon vanilla extract

¼ teaspoon ground cinnamon (optional)
¼ teaspoon sea salt (optional)
¼ cup water, or more as needed

Process the avocado, maple syrup, cocoa powder, vanilla, cinnamon, if using, and sea salt in a food processor or high-speed blender. Add the water, as needed, to achieve a smooth mixture.

Pour into glasses and chill, or serve immediately.

Variations: If you don't like cinnamon, do not add it. Or, instead of cinnamon add a drop of mint extract. Or add a pinch of cayenne for some heat!

Bittersweet Chocolate Truffles

By Fran Costigan

Fran Costigan, one of the premier plant-based dessert chefs in the world, made the chocolate wedding cake for Jill and me in 2006. When I was in New York City to host a screening of the movie *Forks Over Knives*, Fran served these E2-friendly, melt-in-your mouth, intensely chocolate truffles and I immediately knew I wanted them in my next book. Fran simply replaced the heavy cream and butter used in traditional truffles with unsweetened soy or almond milk, and used a high cocoa percentage, low-sugar chocolate. And guess what? These taste better! Thanks, Fran.

Prep time: 10 minutes • Cooling time: 3 hours • Makes 30 to 40 round truffles

GANACHE

    8 ounces 70 to 78 percent dark chocolate (bar, not chips!)
    ¾ cup unsweetened soy milk or almond milk
    1½ teaspoons pure vanilla extract

TRUFFLES

    ½ cup unsweetened sifted cocoa powder, for dusting

To make the ganache: On a dry cutting board with a sharp knife, or in a food processor, chop the chocolate finely: the chocolate must be finely chopped so it melts evenly. Transfer the finely chopped chocolate to a glass or metal 3- or 4-cup mixing bowl.

In a small saucepan over medium heat, bring the non-dairy milk to a gentle boil. When you see bubbles around the sides, remove the pan from the heat and add the vanilla extract. Wait 30 seconds and test a few drops of the hot milk on your wrist—it should feel very hot but not scalding. While at this temperature, pour the almond milk and vanilla, *all at once*, over the chocolate in the bowl. Mix gently with a whisk, from the center out, only until the mixture, now called ganache, is perfectly smooth. If you mix too much, the ganache might become grainy.

Pour the ganache into a shallow dish such as a pie plate and press a piece of parchment paper or plastic wrap directly on the surface. Refrigerate until it is no longer liquid, typically 2 to 3 hours. The ganache can be refrigerated at this point for up to 3 days.

When the ganache is very firm, make the truffles: Sift the cocoa powder through a metal strainer into a shallow bowl. Use one spoon to scoop out ¾-inch pieces of the ganache, and another to push the ganache off the spoon into the cocoa powder.

When a dozen or so pieces are made, roll them in the palms of your hands to shape into irregular rounds, then roll in the cocoa powder until coated. Repeat until all of the truffles are made.

To store and serve the truffles: Place the truffles in a single layer into a covered container, separating them with parchment or wax paper. Refrigerate for up to 1 week, or freeze for up to 1 month. The extra cocoa powder coating will keep the truffles separate.

Allow 15 to 20 minutes for the truffles to come to room temperature before serving.

Variation: Gingery Truffles

Add 1½ tablespoons of ground ginger to the cocoa powder. Dust the truffles following the directions for making the truffles (above). Taste a small one, and add more ground ginger if you like yours hot and spicy.

Sprinkle the truffles with a pinch of ground ginger just before serving.

Damn Good Cookies

By Jane Esselstyn

Raw dough, baby! Who isn't in the mood for it sometimes? Jane served this at a Plant-Strong Women, Power, Sex, and Food presentation and everyone loved it, right down to the very last spoonful! You will, too. Like revenge, we find this is a dish best served cold.

Prep time: 5 minutes • Makes 20 teaspoon-size cookies

½ cup raw almonds (or raw cashews)

½ cup raw walnuts

6 large dates, pitted

1 tablespoon vanilla extract

1 tablespoon water (if needed for texture)

Pinch of sea salt (optional)

3 tablespoons no-dairy-added, dark chocolate chips

3 tablespoons old-fashioned oats

1 tablespoon water (if needed for texture)

In a food processor or high-speed blender, blend the nuts until crumbled uniformly. Transfer the nut mixture to a bowl, and set aside.

Add the dates, vanilla, and water to the food processor or high-speed blender, and blend until the mixture is paste-like. Scrape down the sides of the processor bowl or blender jar a few times, if needed, and blend again.

Add the reserved nut mixture to the date mixture and blend together. Add the chocolate chips and oats and pulse the mixture until blended to your liking, or mix in the chips and oats by hand, if you prefer.

Press balls of the mixture firmly into a teaspoon. Free the dough from the spoon's shape and place on a serving plate.

Serve immediately—if you can't help yourself—otherwise chill first.

Acknowledgments

I want to thank and acknowledge the many people who helped make this book possible. First, Grand Central Publishing for deciding to go another round with me and helping to spread the plant-strong message. Specifically, I would like to thank Diana Baroni, Matthew Ballast, and Jamie Raab. I would like to thank my literary agent, Richard Pine with Inkwell Management, for plucking me out of relative obscurity and sending me off on a purpose-driven life. I would like to thank Whole Foods Market and the remarkable John Mackey for giving me the opportunity to partner with them as they bravely and boldly go where no supermarket has gone before.

I would like to thank the individual members of the Engine 2 team who are in it to win it with me every single day and are slugging it out helping people rescue their health with something as simple as food: Dani Little, the stalwart, competent, and always consistent Engine 2 program director; Natala Constantine, the Engine 2 social media guru who does the work of five people; Jillian Gibson, the always upbeat event manager with the Health Talent Group; Mike Schall and Mike McKeon and their unwavering commitment to the Engine 2, Plant-Strong food line; and Adam Reiser, the principal of the Health Talent Group who has helped me steer and navigate Engine 2 to become all that it is today. I would like to thank the amazing evolutionary psychologist Doug Lisle for his guidance and brilliance with E2 retreats, business, and this book. I would like to thank my buddy and nutritionist extraordinaire Jeff Novick for sharing his knowledge and time with this book, Engine 2 Immersion retreats, and life. I would like to thank Christopher McDougall, Brandon Brazier, and Scott Jurek for their time and interviews for this book, and Miranda Spencer, Nick Bromley, and Ted Tetsuhiko for their help with research and editing. I would like to thank Jaidev Shergill for speaking his mind with such clarity and charm. It touched me and the book to the core. I would like to thank my parents,

Ann and Essy, for giving me a lifelong foundation of support, enthusiasm, and encouragement to unflinchingly always say "yes" to life. I would like to thank my siblings and their spouses—Ted and Anne, Zeb and Polly, and Jane and Brian—for their interest, curiosity, and counseling on all things Engine 2.

I would like to thank my nieces and nephews who jumped in and helped with the Engine 2 retreats: Crile, Zeb, Bainon, Flinn, Gus, and Rose. I would like to give a huge call out and extra, extra special thank you to my sister, Jane, who tore into the recipe section with an unbridled amount of boldness and braveness and has created a masterpiece of plant-strong goodness for people all over the world. You nailed it, Jane!

I also want to thank my sensei and co-writer of *The Engine 2 Diet* and this book, Gene Stone. We did it, Gener! Plants rule and you rule! Whoever would have thought we could bring *My Beef with Meat* back from the ashes. "You never know. You just never know."

Lastly, I would like to thank my family: my wife, Jill; my son, Kole; my daughter, Sophie; and the gentlemanly Tug. You all have made huge sacrifices on behalf of Engine 2 as we steer people towards a lighter, healthier, and happier life. Sophie, I want to thank you for always wanting to "share a grapefruit" with me. Kole, I want to thank you for always wanting to go for a bike ride or a swim, or just hang with me. Tug, I want to thank you for your smile, your joy, your loyalty, and our evening walks. And Jill, I want to thank you for always having my back and for keeping me grounded. I love you all to the moon and back.

Index

About the Author

RIP ESSELSTYN was born in upstate New York, raised in Cleveland, Ohio, and educated at the University of Texas at Austin, where he was a three-time All-American swimmer. After graduation Rip spent a decade as one of the premier triathletes in the world. He then joined the Austin Fire Department, where he introduced his passion for a whole-food, plant-based diet to Austin's Engine 2 Firehouse in order to rescue a firefighting brother's health. To document his success he wrote the national best-selling book *The Engine 2 Diet*, which shows the irrefutable connection between a plant-based diet and good health.

Recently Rip left his job as a firefighter to team up with Whole Foods Market as one of their Healthy Eating Partners to raise awareness for Whole Foods employees, customers, and communities about the benefits of eating a plant-strong diet. He has appeared on hundreds of radio shows as well as national television shows, including the *Today* show, the CBS *Sunday Morning* show, *Good Morning America*, and *The Dr. Oz Show*.

Rip lives in Austin, Texas, with his wife, Jill Kolasinski, and their two beautiful children, Kole and Sophie.